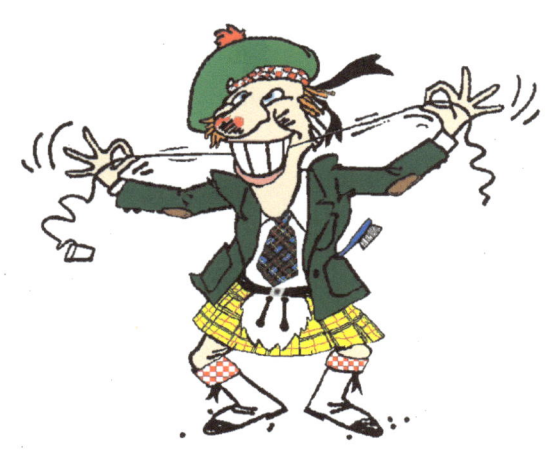

# The Practice Book

### Dentistry That Lasts - Quality That Counts

*The Practice Book*
Written and produced by Neil Stewart McLeod
Los Angeles
May 2015

*By the same author*

One for the Pot
A Ship In A Bottle
The Aching Heart
Pure Whimsy
My Silver Box
When the Spirit Moves
The Clan Remembers
A Cartload of Stories
The Persimmon Tree
The Thorn With Me
Songs and Poems of Frances McLeod
The Illustrated Address To A Haggis
Letters From A Scottish Chief
Bringing the Clan Back to Dunvegan
Dental Ditties
Another Cuppa
Upon Reflection
Nearly Jewish
An Editor's Corner
Christmas Poems

Cover Images - crests of the University of Southern California, London University, Guys Hospital, Royal College of Surgeons, Beverly Hills Acdemy of Dentistry, Pacific Coast Society for Prosthodontics, The Los Angeles Dental Society and Dr. McLeod's invention the Contact Marker.

ISBN-13: 978-1514103487

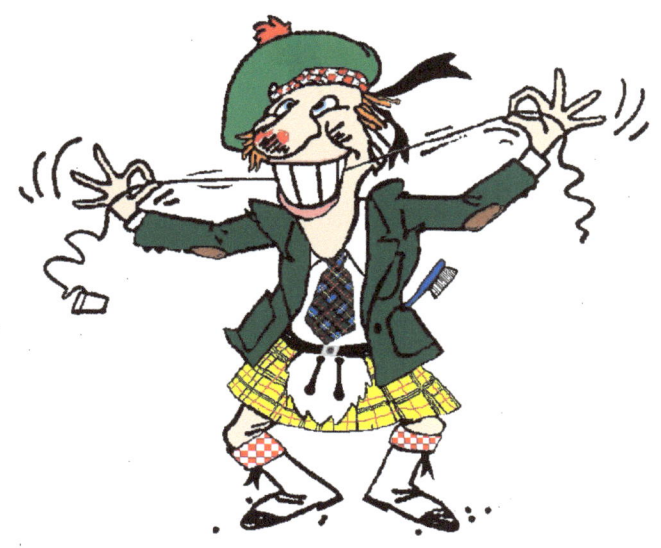

# The Practice Book

Dentistry That Lasts - Quality That Counts

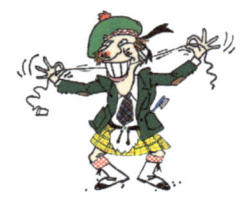

# D.D.S. On The Door

D.D.S. on the door which you enter
A painless and shiny adventure,
Your mouth might be
A licorice factory,
But you sure as hell don't want no denture.

His chairs are as comfy as a tub
And his girls show you just where to scrub,
Enthusiasm bubbling,
With bristles for scrubbing,
At Neil McLeod's Plaque Control Club.

Oh yes my friend as of today
You'll notice decline of decay,
Soon you'll be dating
'Stead of waiting room waiting,
Neil McLeod real McCoy I'll say.

*by Hans VanVeen*

# Contents

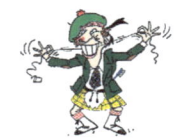

# A Brief History of The Practice

Dr. Earl Pound, renowned researcher, clinician and lecturer of complete denture esthetics and function, graduated from the University of Southern California School of Dentistry in 1923. He immediately opened an entertainment practice in Hollywood. In 1929 Dr. Coryden Glazier graduated from U.S.C. and joined the practice. Dr. Glazier became president of the Gold Foil Study Club at USC, and president of the Hollywood Dental Society. When America joined the war in 1941, Dr. Pound joined the Navy and subsequently pursued his academic career. Dr. Glazier continued as principle of the practice and moved it from Hollywood and Highland to the newly erected medical building at Sunset and Doheny. Dr. Neil McLeod, also a U.S.C. graduate, took over the practice in September of 1976 which still continues, and is now one of the oldest dental practices in Los Angeles. Dr. McLeod was president of the Beverly Hills Academy of Dentistry, and has lectured of precision attachments and web presence for dentists. Like Dr. Pound, Dr. McLeod enjoyed membership in the Pacific Coast Society for Prosthodontics.

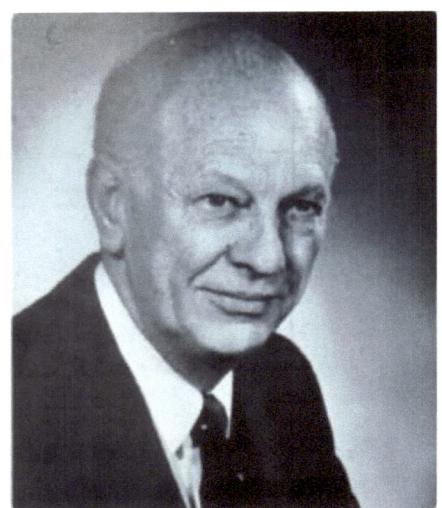
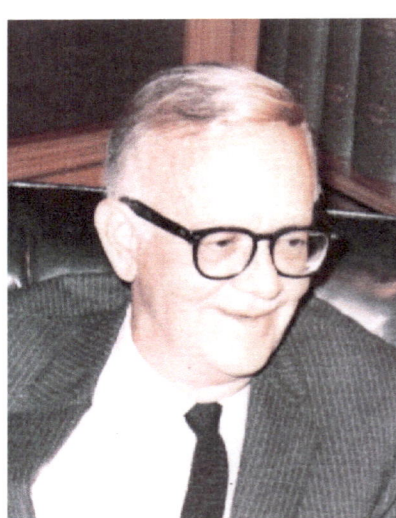
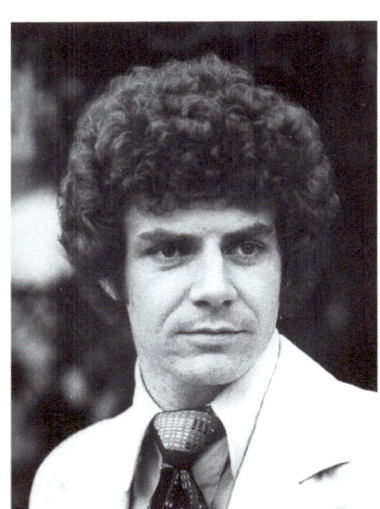

*Dr. Earl Pound 1950's*     *Dr. Coryden Glazier 1969*     *Dr. Neil McLeod 1976*

# Practice Philosophy

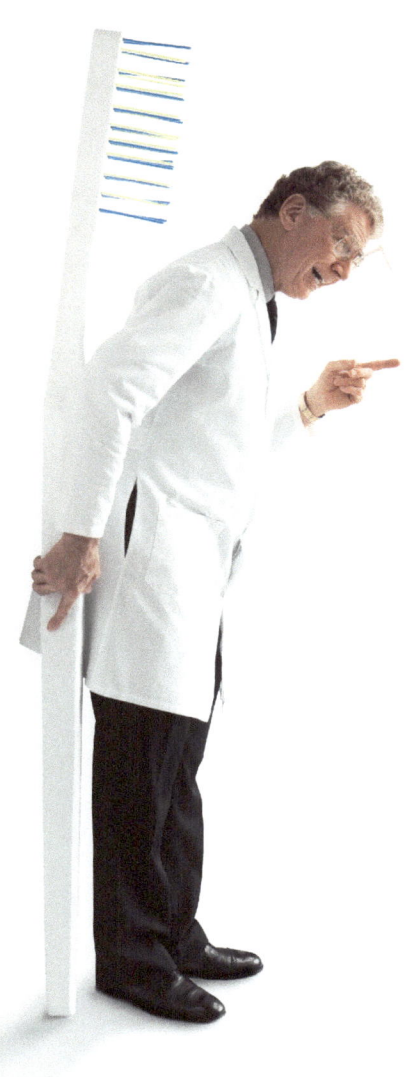

The emphasis is always on the quality of care. In a practice that is over ninety years old, with some patients who are now over ninety years of age, it is easy for us to be able to see what type of dentistry lasts. Only high quality care that can be shown to be of lasting value is provided.

### Education & Prevention
As a practice, we are true believers that preventative care and education are the keys to optimal dental health. We strive to provide "dental health care" vs. "disease care". That's why we focus on thorough exams – checking the overall health of your teeth and gums, performing oral cancer exams, and taking x-rays when necessary. We also know that routine cleanings, flossing, sealants, and fluoride are all helpful in preventing dental disease. Not only are we focused on the beauty of your smile, we're also concerned about your health. A review of your medical history can help us stay informed of your overall health, any new medications, and any illnesses that may impact your dental health.

### Training & Expertise
As your dental health professionals, we want you to be confident knowing that we are a team of highly trained and skilled clinicians. We pride ourselves in providing the care you need to keep your smile healthy. To give you the best possible service and results, we are committed to continual education and learning. We attend dental lectures, meetings, and dental conventions to stay informed of new techniques, the latest products, and the newest equipment that a modern dental office can utilize to provide state-of-the-art dental care. Also, being members of various professional dental associations helps us to stay abreast of the changes and recommendations for our profession.

### A Positive Experience
Building a foundation of trust by treating our patients as special individuals is vital to our success. We understand how uneasy some patients may feel about their dental visits, and how we can make a difference in providing a relaxing and positive experience. Our entire team is dedicated to providing you with excellent, personalized care and service to make your visits as comfortable and pleasant as possible.

*Photo by David Blattel*

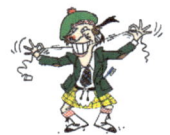

4

# Announcements

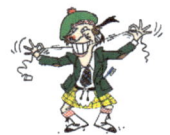

*9201 Sunset Boulevard*

**CORYDON J. GLAZIER, D.D.S.**

9201 Sunset Boulevard, Suite 715

Los Angeles, California 90069

275-5379

Dear

After 50 years of general practice, I am retiring September

1, 1976. I want to express my deep appreciation for having

had the privilege of serving you in the past.

I strongly recommend that you continue your dental main-

tenance with my successor, Dr. Neil Stewart McLeod, a U.S.C.

graduate. You will find him to be a compassionate, highly

qualified and experienced dentist who is fully acquainted with

your dental history.

My very best wishes

*Corydon J. Glazier D.D.S.*

C. J. Glazier, D.D.S.

**NEIL STEWART McLEOD**

B.D.S. (LOND.), L.D.S. R.C.S. (ENG.), D.D.S.

ANNOUNCES THE OPENING OF HIS OFFICE AT

**THE BEVERLY SUNSET MEDICAL CENTER**

**9201 SUNSET BOULEVARD, SUITE 715**

**LOS ANGELES, CALIFORNIA 90069**

WHERE HE PRACTICES GENERAL DENTISTRY

———

BY APPOINTMENT                    (213) 275-5379

# Dentistry That Lasts - Quality That Counts

# Services

The offices are located at 9201 Sunset Boulevard at Doheny Road at the edge of Beverly Hills, in the Sunset Medical Tower. Easy parking is available in the building, and city transport services stop right outside.

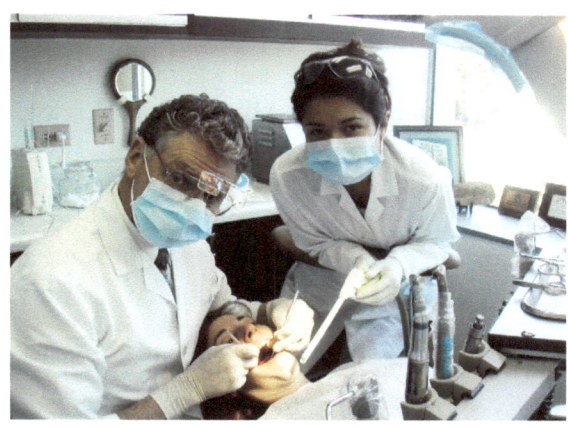

We have a team of expert dental specialists with whom we work closely. We are a dental practice devoted to restoring and enhancing the natural beauty of your teeth using conservative, state-of-the-art procedures that will result in beautiful, long lasting smiles!

Whether it is for complete dental care or a second opinion, an implant to support a replacement tooth or just a simple filling, treat yourself to the comfort of knowing how to preserve your "Biting chance at life".

**High Standards**

A standard of excellence in personalized dental care enables us to provide the quality dental services our patients deserve. We provide comprehensive treatment planning and use restorative and cosmetic dentistry to achieve your optimal dental health. Should a dental emergency occur, we make every effort to see and care for you as soon as possible.

**Uncompromising Safety**

Infection control in our office is also very important to us. To protect our patients and ourselves, we strictly maintain sterilization and cross contamination processes using standards that meet or exceed those recommended by the American Dental Association (ADA), the Occupational Safety and Health Administration (OSHA), and the Center for Disease Control (CDC).

We thank you for allowing us to take care of your dental needs and look forward to serving you.

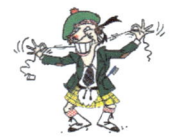

# Meet the Doctor

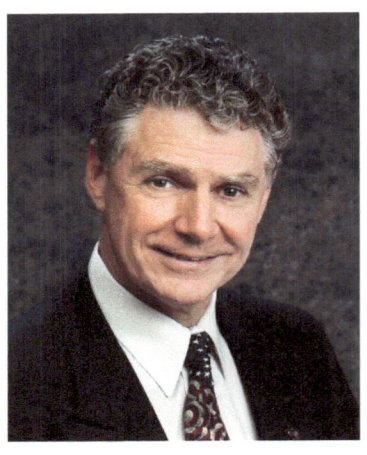

Doctor McLeod is a USC Dental School graduate who has been a practicing dentist since 1972, and has worked both in London and Los Angeles. In his final year at Guy's Hospital Dental School he was a recipient of the Alfred Rycroft Traveling Scholarship to Tufts University Dental School in Boston. After graduating from Guy's Hospital Dental School, he continued in hospital service there while working for his primary fellowship in the Royal College of Surgeons. In 1974 he came to the United States on a Fulbright Scholarship to study at the University of Southern California.

On completing his training, Doctor McLeod acquired an established Hollywood practice in 1976 where he specializes in restorative and preventive dentistry. The focus is on high quality work that lasts, and on helping the patients prevent dental disease. His research, lectures and publications on semi precision and precision retainers gained him acceptance and membership in the Pacific Coast Society for Prosthodontics.

Dr. McLeod was born in Oxford, England, and raised in the British colony of Kenya in East Africa. Among his professional associations, are memberships in the International Academy of Gnathology and the Academy of General Dentistry. Dr. McLeod's articles on precision attachments have been published in the Journal of Prosthetic Dentistry. He has written and appeared in forty television information spots, and has made numerous radio and television appearances on a number of issues including dentistry. Doctor McLeod has served as a Consumer Advisor for the American Dental Association.

In Doctor McLeod's dental practice they specialize in fine reconstructive and preventative dental care. The emphasis is on communication with the patients so that they may make informed decisions about how their mouths are to be treated, and what types of materials are used to repair the teeth. This uncompromising commitment to proper care has shown itself to be of long lasting value, and undeniable success, especially when reviewing the treatment of patients who are senior citizens, and for whom the dentistry is still lasting decades after it was installed.

**Give yourself a Biting chance at life**

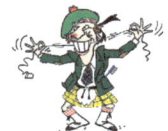

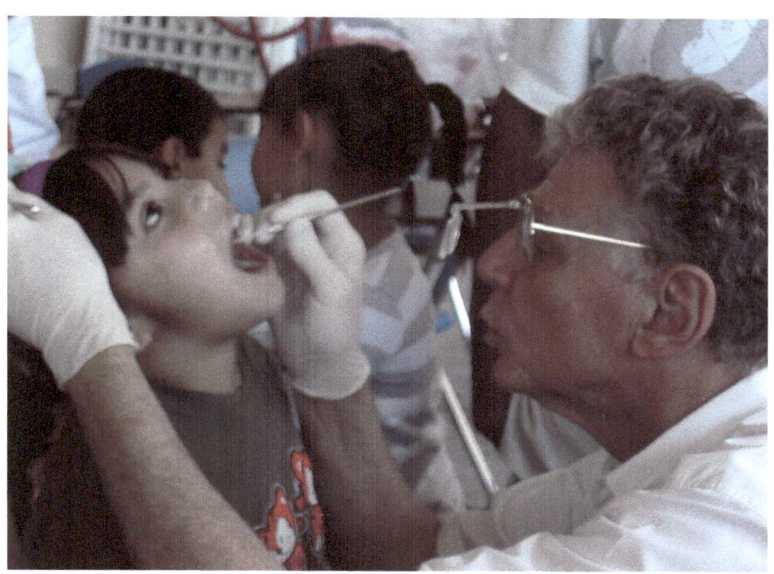

Volunteering at the Hogar Orphanage brings skilled diagnostic training to the needy where it can be of great value, to the young as they grow and develop. The interest and curiosity of these little ones is disarming.

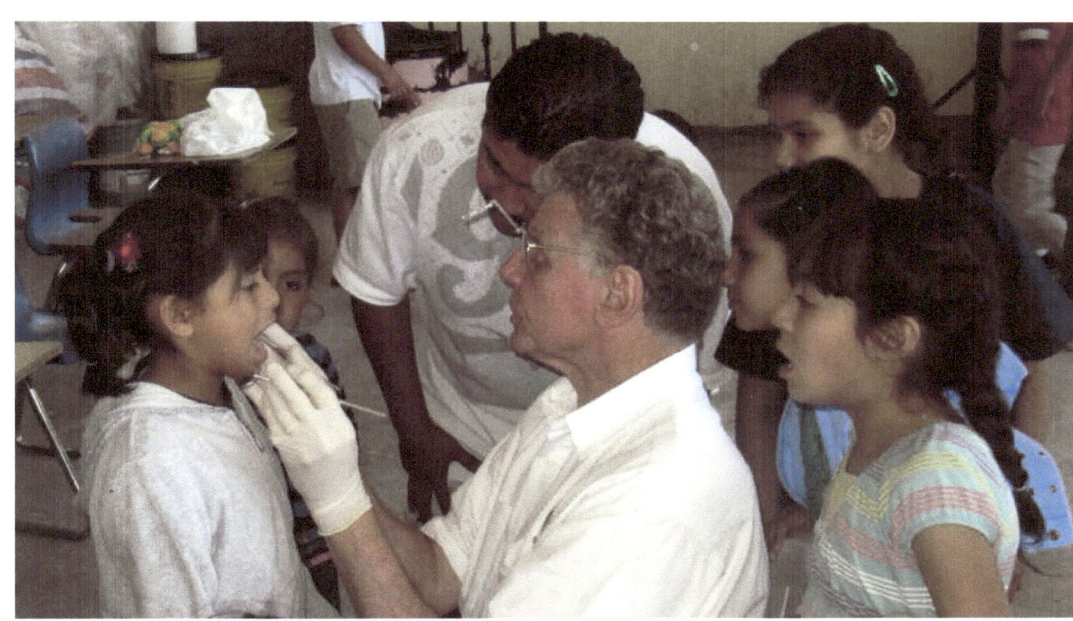

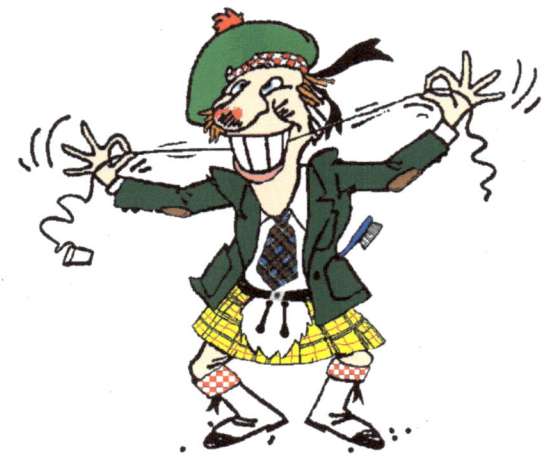

*Phil MaCavity says "Just Floss 'em"!*

# About Phil The Practice Logo

Phil MaCavity has been the practice logo since the late 1970's, and with a slogan of - *Phil MacCavity says "Just Floss 'em".*- it has been a very successful and popular icon. It was drawn by Colin Bailey the illustrator who worked for the Mattel Corporation. He was a patient and friend of the doctor who when asked if he could come up with a drawing of a flossing Scot dancing a jig immediately asked, "Ah now! Do you want him wearing a Glengarry or a Balmoral, and what about those leather patches on the elbows and horn buttons?" Within a few days a selection of drawings arrived one of which you see here.

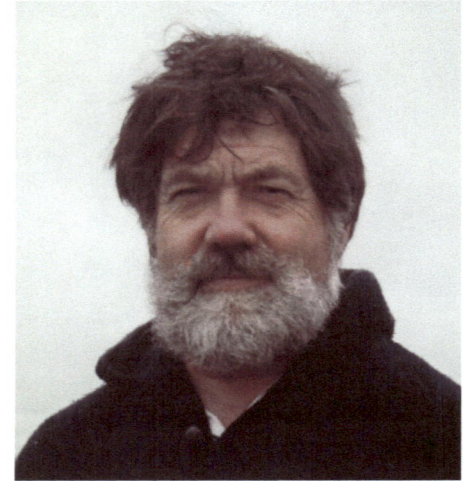

*Colin Bailey*

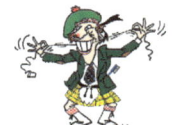

# Dental Cleanings
# Pocket Measurements and Gum Treatments

You must have your teeth professionally cleaned regularly. They will deteriorate if you don't. Our highly trained staff can help you. Measuring the depths of your "gum" pockets provides essential information about the structures supporting your teeth.

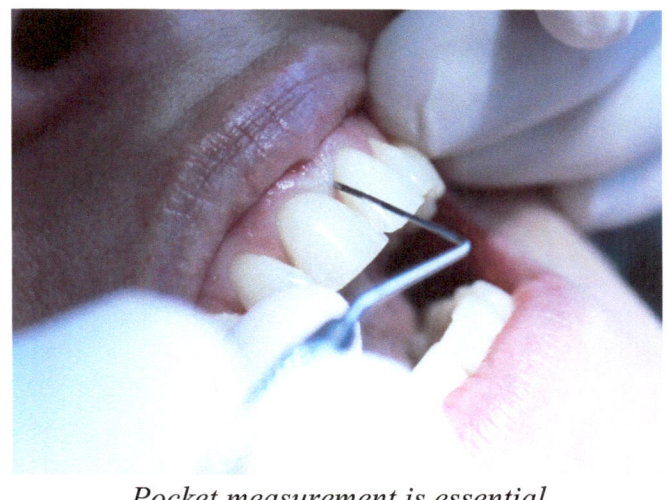

*Pocket measurement is essential*

## For Not Flossing

To Beelzebub and his chums
Go all those who won't floss, the bums,
Now they're wailing and weeping
And flaying and leaping
And gnashing away on their gums.

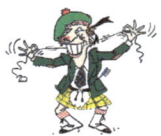

# Flossing

In her 1798 letter to Admiral Lord Nelson, shortly before he left for the battle of the Nile, Lady Hamilton wrote, "Don't forget to pack your dental twine dear!" Nelson returned victorious though minus an arm and many of his teeth. Clearly the upper echelons of society knew the value of using fine string to clean between the teeth. Everyone should now be flossing.

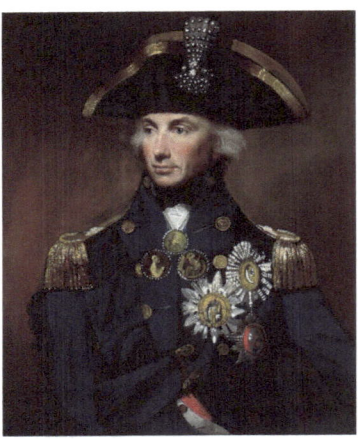

*Admiral Lord Nelson* Public Domain

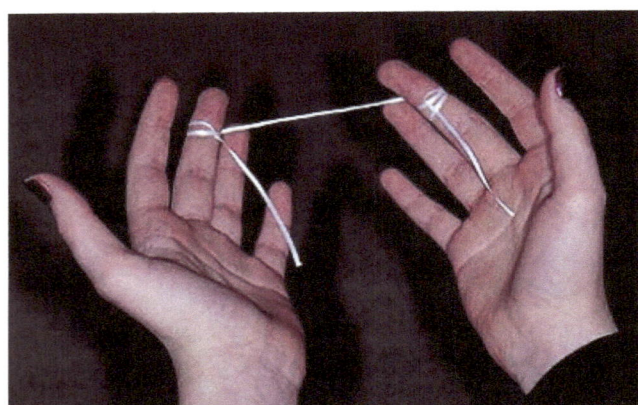

We teach all our patients to floss properly. This is a manual skill which needs to be practiced and perfected by everyone.
You don't have to floss all your teeth, just the ones you want to keep

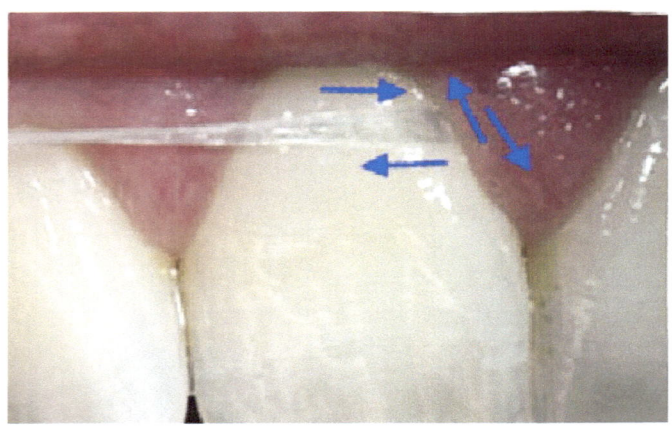

## A Lot of Rot

If flossing your teeth night and day
Is causing your fingers to fray
You might choose not to care
What happens in there
And just let your teeth rot away .

# Cancer Screening

We check for changes in the tissues of the mouth which may become life threatening.

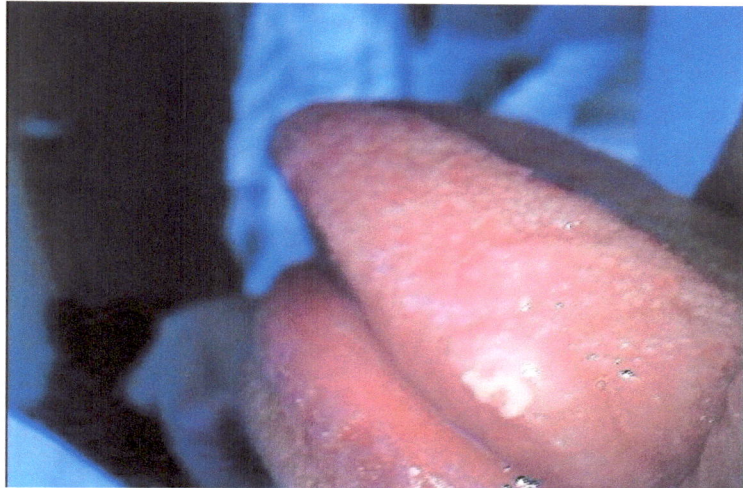

*Leukoplakia - white pre-cancerous change on tongue*

Doctor McLeod
Tells you out loud
To open your mouth
Very "widee."
So you open your jaws,
And you do this because
He needs to see
What is "insidee!"

*Myra Friedman*
*January 2015*

Detected early the survival rate of oral cancer can be over 80%, but left late, and after six months, the mortality rate can be that high. Tobacco products, alcohol, hot food, spicy food and repeated trauma all cause oral cancer as does Human Papilloma Virus. It is essential that tissue changes be detected early to prevent drastic treatments or mortality. Regular examinations not further than six months apart is therefore ideal.

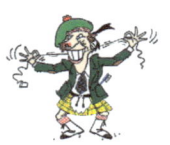

# X-rays and Diagnosis

Dental x-rays may reveal, abscesses or cysts, bone loss, cancerous and non-cancerous tumors, decay between the teeth, developmental abnormalities, poor tooth and root positions, problems inside a tooth or below the gum line, the presence of bone and fractures. They are an essential diagnostic tool which we use to plan your treatment.

Detecting and treating dental problems at an early stage may save you time, money and unnecessary discomfort. The new digital x-rays decrease the radiation dosage by nearly 90%. We like to see new x-rays every three years routinely, and when necessary to diagnose.

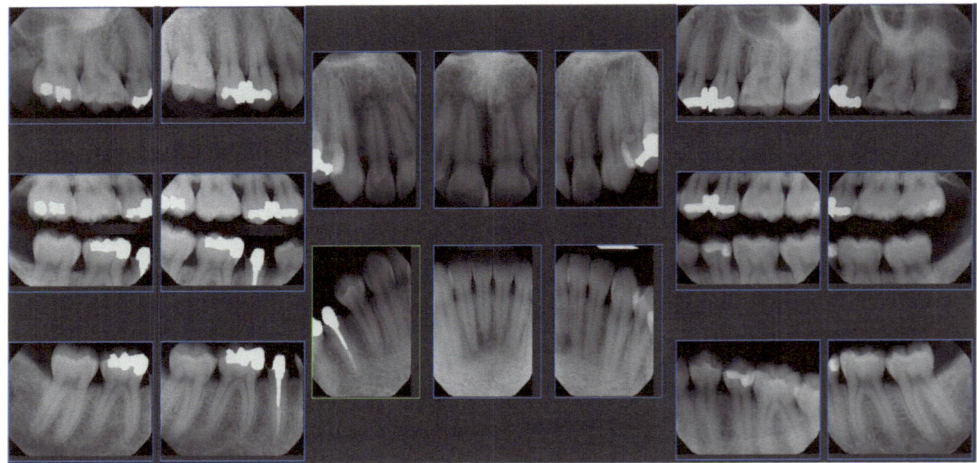

These images give us astonishing amounts of information.

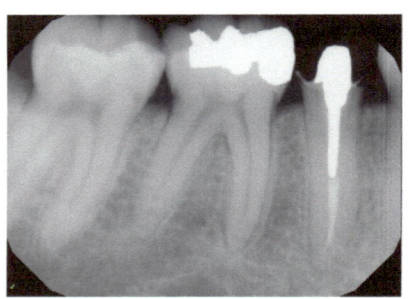

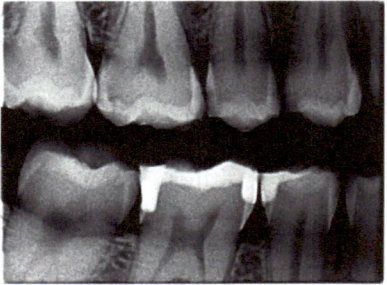

There's a mannie I ken, he's a poet
He's dentist and also a Scot
But unless you follow his direction
Your teeth will fall out with the rot !

*Dermot McQuarrie*

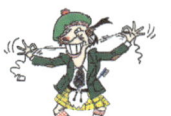

Cat Scans show us in three dimensions where tissues are positioned so that we can plan for implants and diagnose treatment needs.

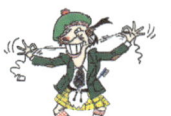

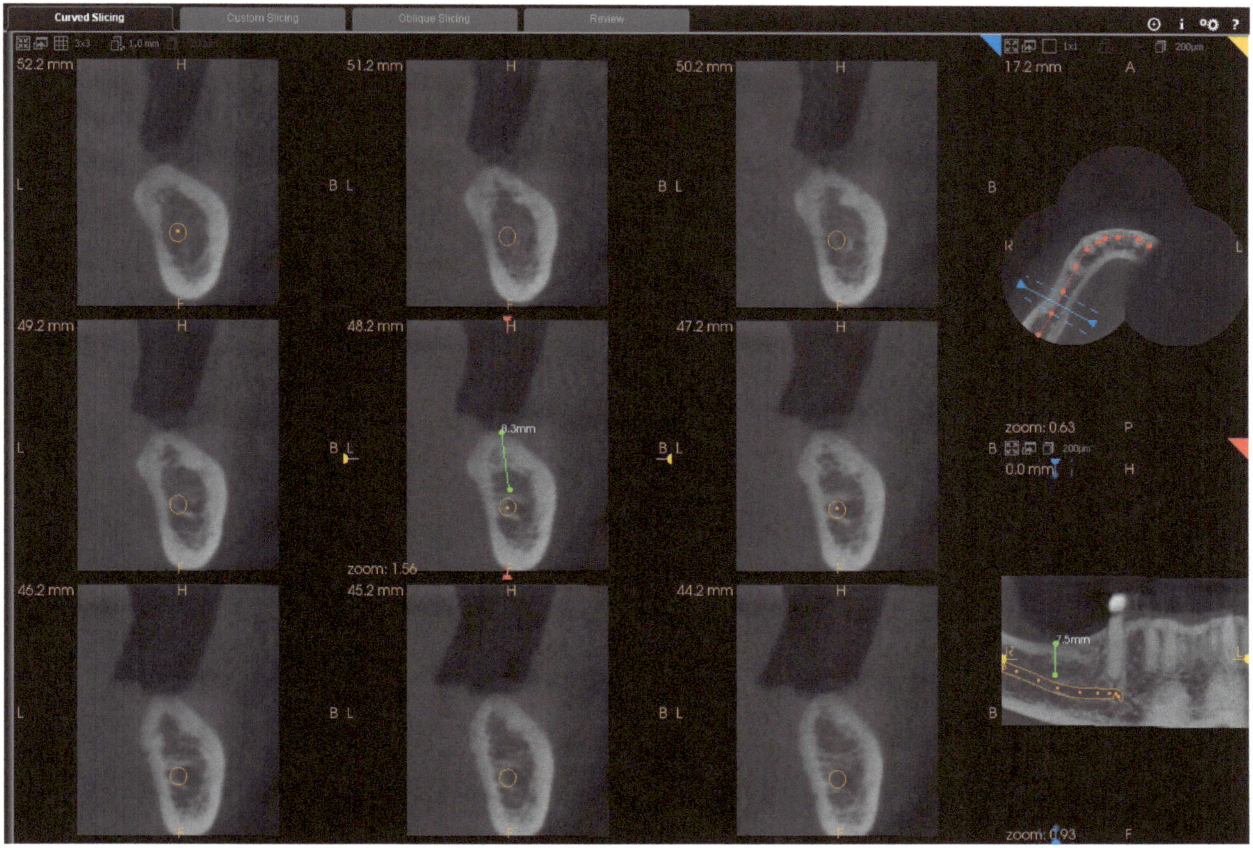

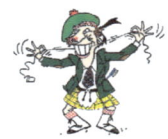

Panelyptical scans are invaluable for a complete overall impression when considering where unerupted teeth lie in the jaw, and the condition of the temporomandibular joints. Wisdom teeth erupt at about the time when youngsters are starting to get a handle on what life is about – sixteen to twenty five, hence "wisdom".

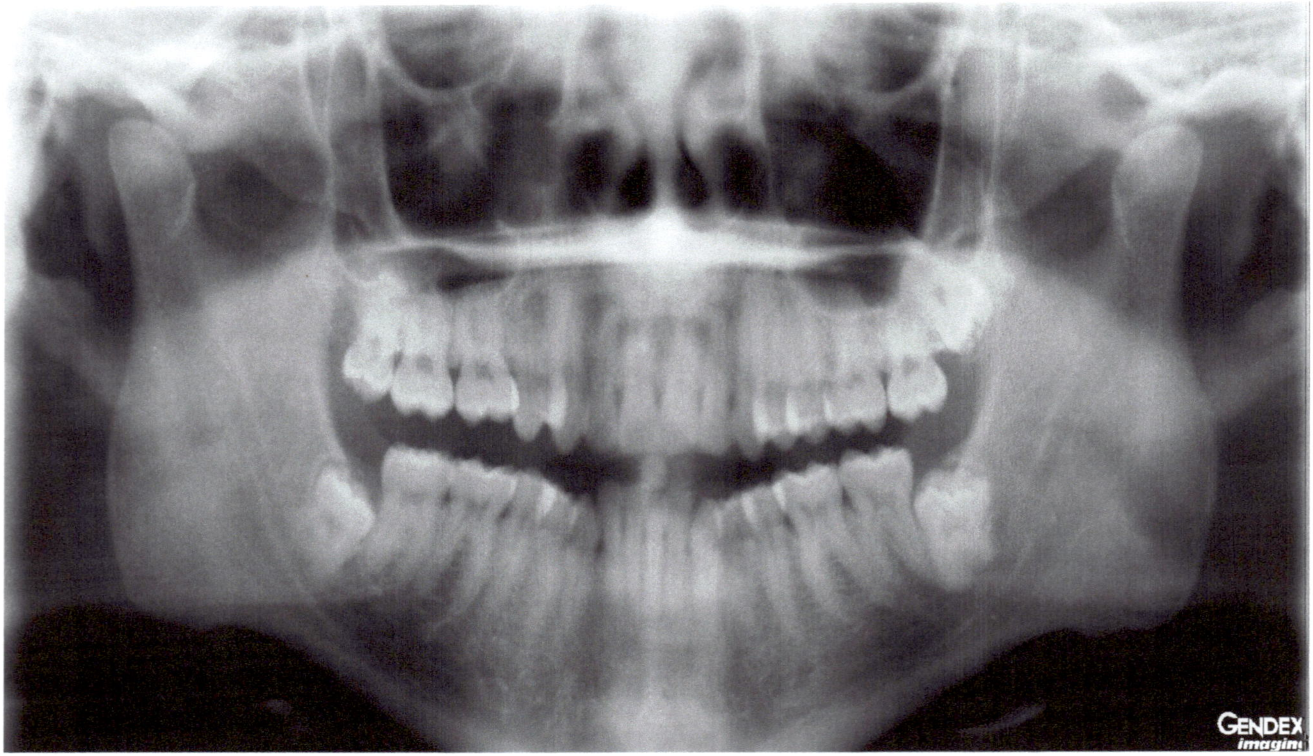

> Wisdom Teeth
> *Haiku*
> When the time is right
> Four extra teeth will appear
> Then you'll be wiser

# Fillings and Inlays

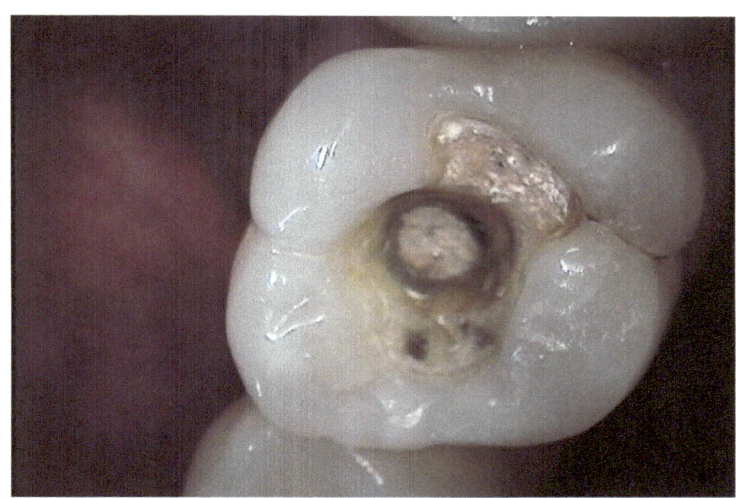

*Cavity in a molar*

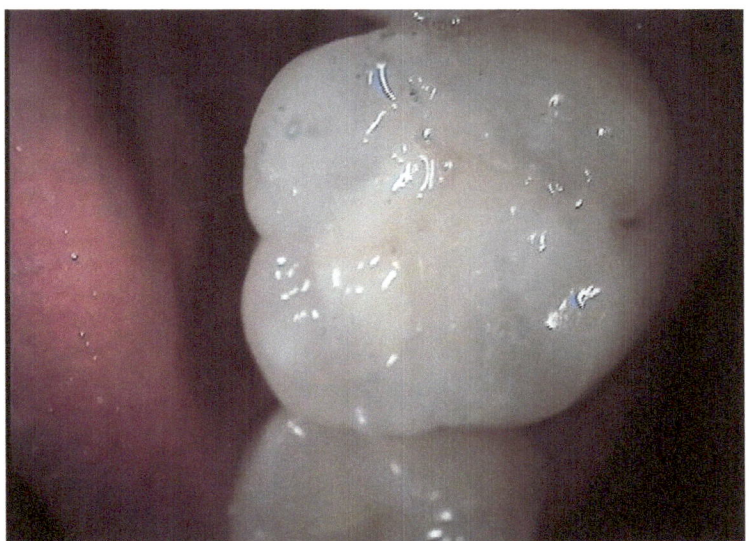

*A porcelain inlay repair*

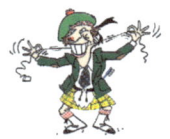

# Gum Grafting

Surgical techniques have now been developed to the point where we can replace receded gum tissue and significantly increase the life of a tooth, and improve the smile. We work with expert Periodontists who provide this service for our patients.

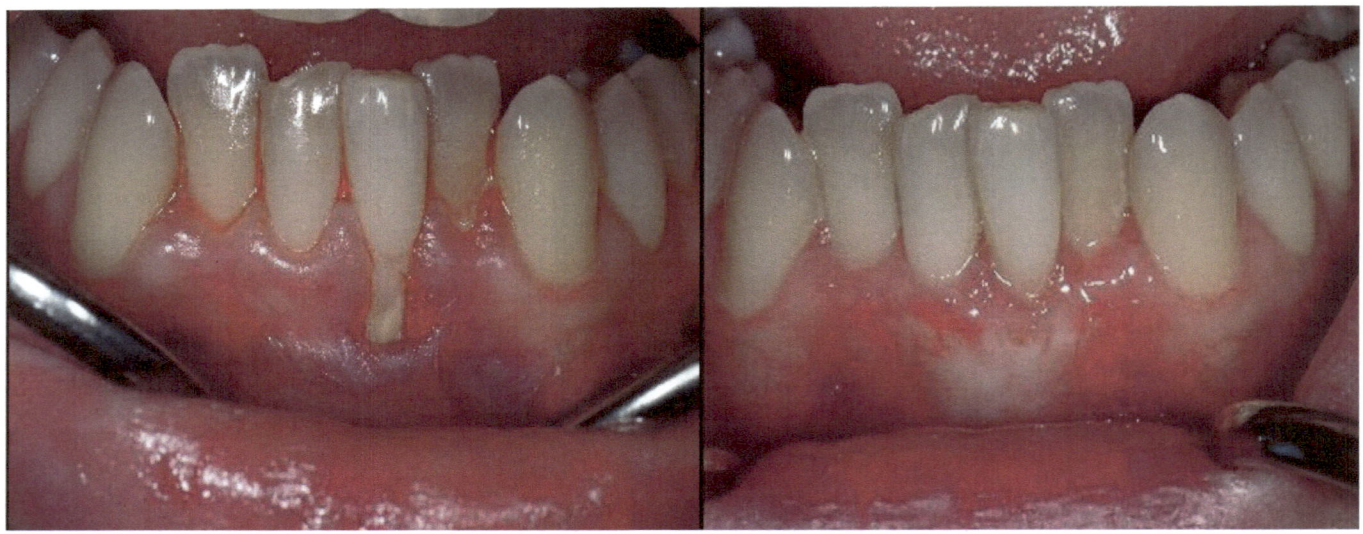

*Graft surgery to eliminate recession and enhance the smile*

*Surgical result by Dr. Sharyar Baradaran*

These exquisite results demonstrate the standard of expert technical support we are able to offer our patients.

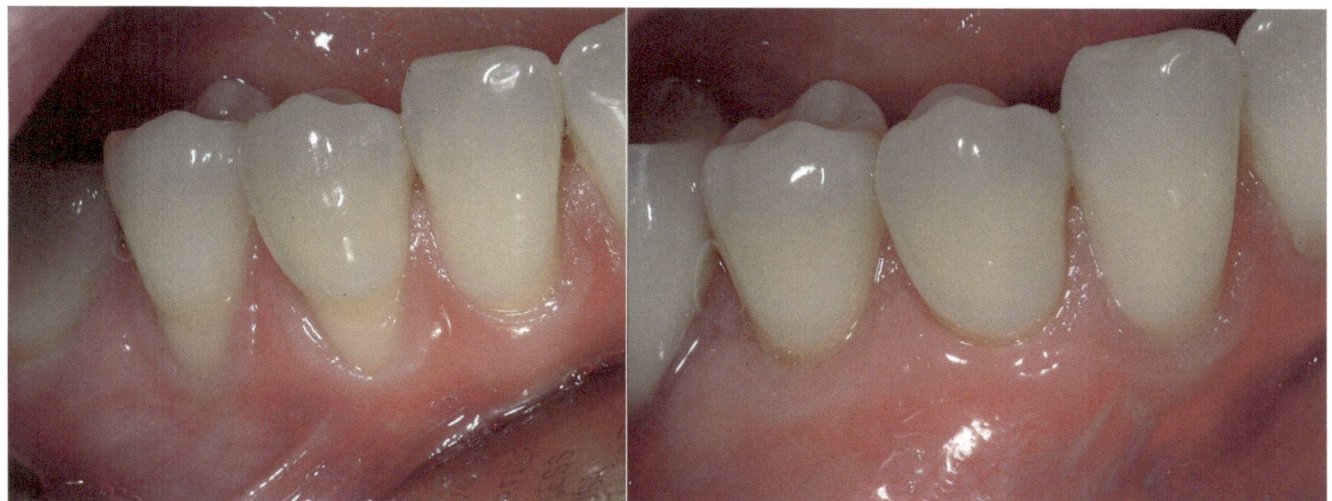

*Surgery for root coverage and improved esthetics*

*Surgical result by Dr. Sharyar Baradaran*

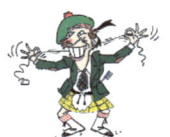

# Onlays and Crowns

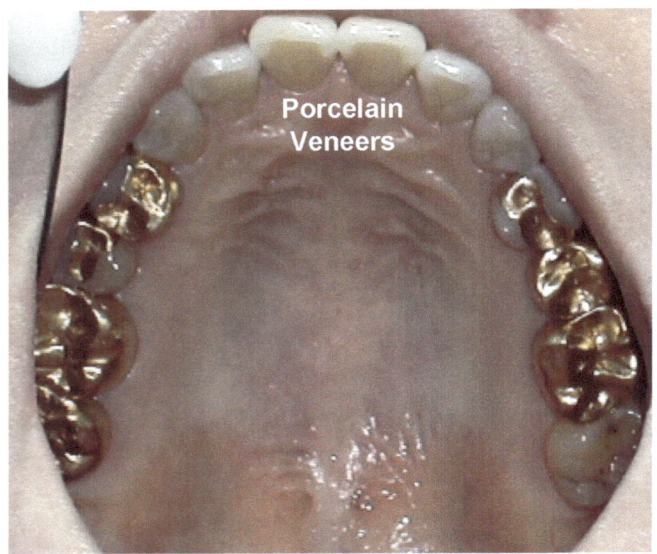

Porcelain Veneers

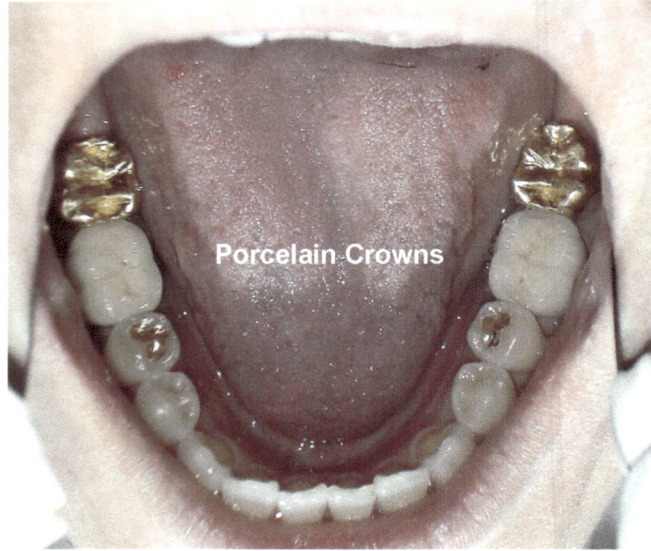

Porcelain Crowns

Crowns and onlays have traditionally been most successfully made of precious metal. Today's revolutionary developments in ceramics allow us to restore teeth with tooth colored materials.

This is an example of a transitional restoration between these two eras. Note the gold onlays and crowns in the upper jaw, and the porcelain veneers on the two upper front teeth and the porcelain crowns on the two lower first molars

---

## Tucker's Gold

*For R. V. Tucker DDS*

A Washington dentist named Tucker
Who made inlays on which folks ate supper
Said, "Fear not if your row
Of teeth show the gold's glow,
When you're smiling just make your lips pucker."

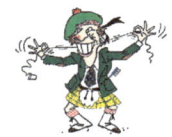

Gold onlays are engineered so that they do not show in the smile, and porcelain veneers are almost imperceptible.

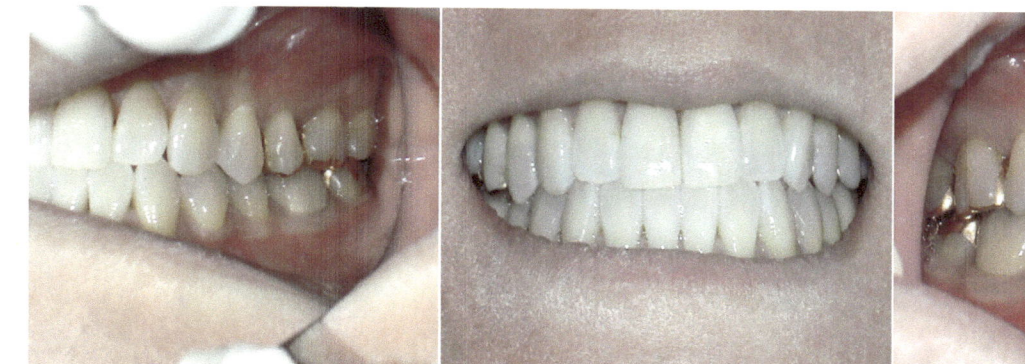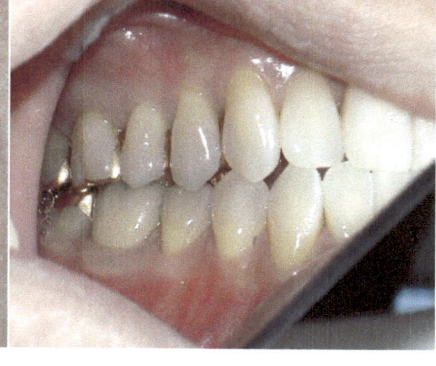

*The same mouth*

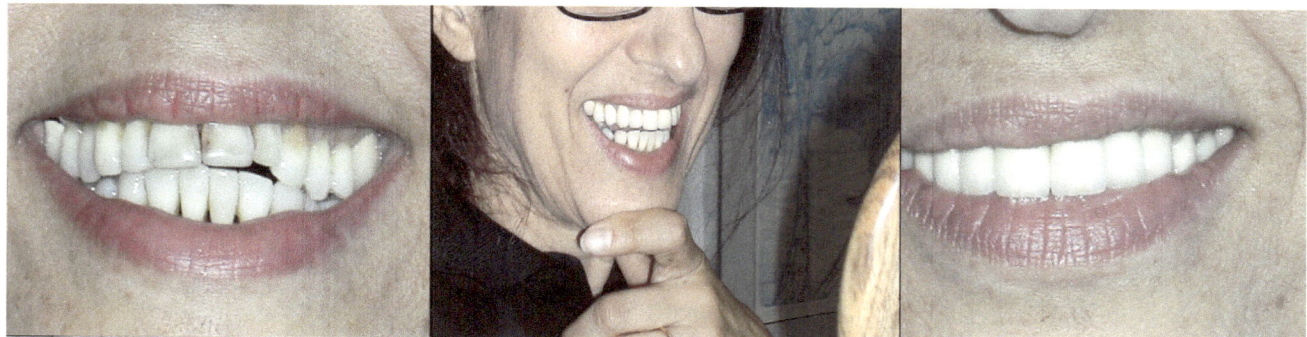

*Crowns transforming a crooked smile*

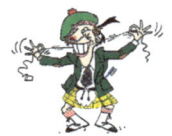

# Temporary Crowns

Ever since the discovery of the polymethyl methacrylate polymer in the 1930's the material has been increasingly used in dentistry. We can now make tooth colored temporary crowns from acrylic and similar polymers so that a patient's appearance can be acceptably maintained while the final laboratory work is being manufactured. Dentistry took an astonishing step forward for our patients.

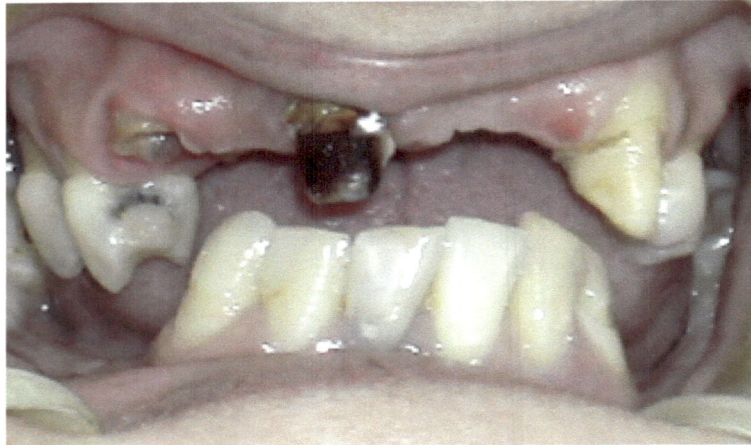

*Urgent need for teeth replacement*

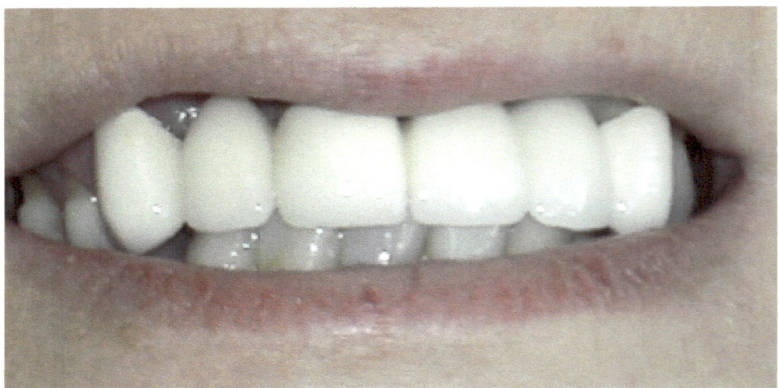

*Immediately placed temporary crowns of acrylic*

# Temporary Cement

The obtundent oil from the clove is used to make a cement which relieves pain and allows ease of removal of temporary crowns.

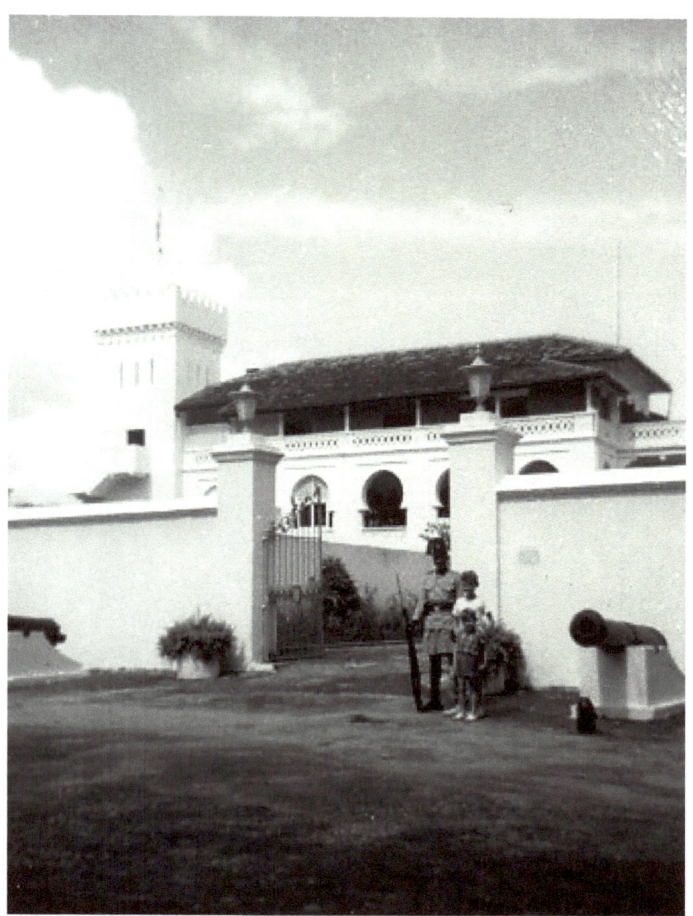

*The author with his brother
at the Sultan's Palace on Zanzibar 1958*

## Cloves

Set in the Indian Ocean,
Off the African coast, but not far,
There's a fertile oasis surrounded by sea-
The Island of Zanzibar.

This mystical tropical haven
Set with palaces, palms and a fort,
Is dotted with trees that bear a spice
Which for centuries long has been sought.

The Caesars had seen it imported,
Though they knew not from whence it came.
They brought it by galley from Palestine
To relieve their dental pain.

This valuable spice was transported
By caravan over the sand,
From a port in the south of Arabia
And by dhow from that far distant land.

The seeds of this spice have a fragrant oil,
An obtundent for which many strove.
We know the oil as Eugenol,
The remarkable spice is the clove.

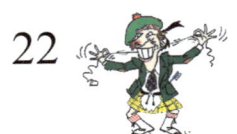

# Porcelain Crowns

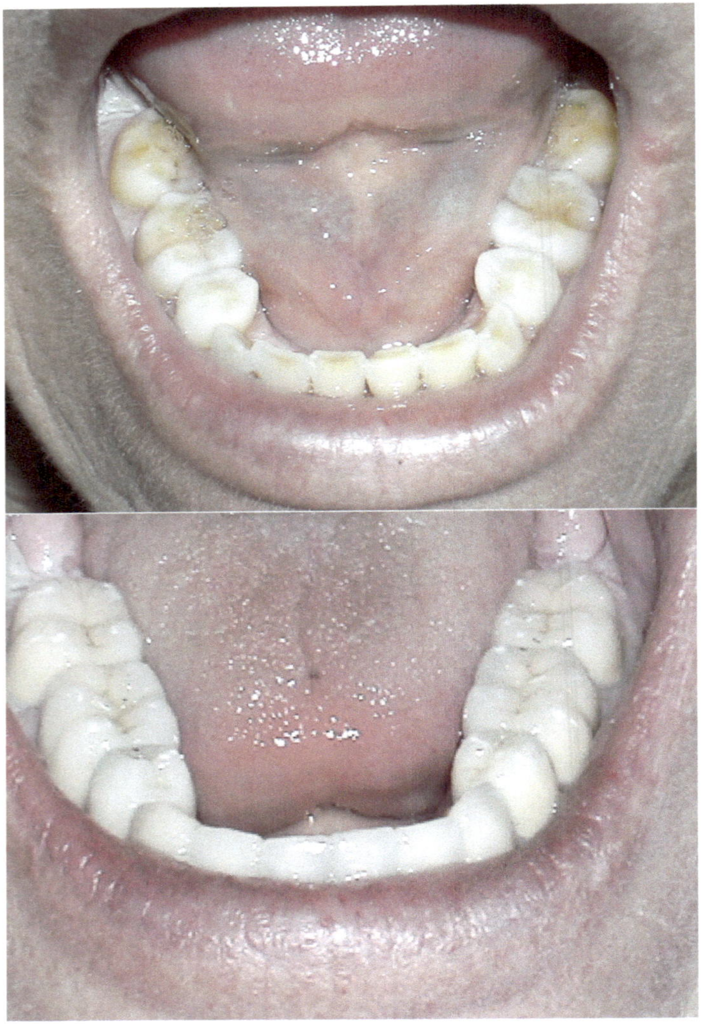

*Seriously eroded teeth restored*

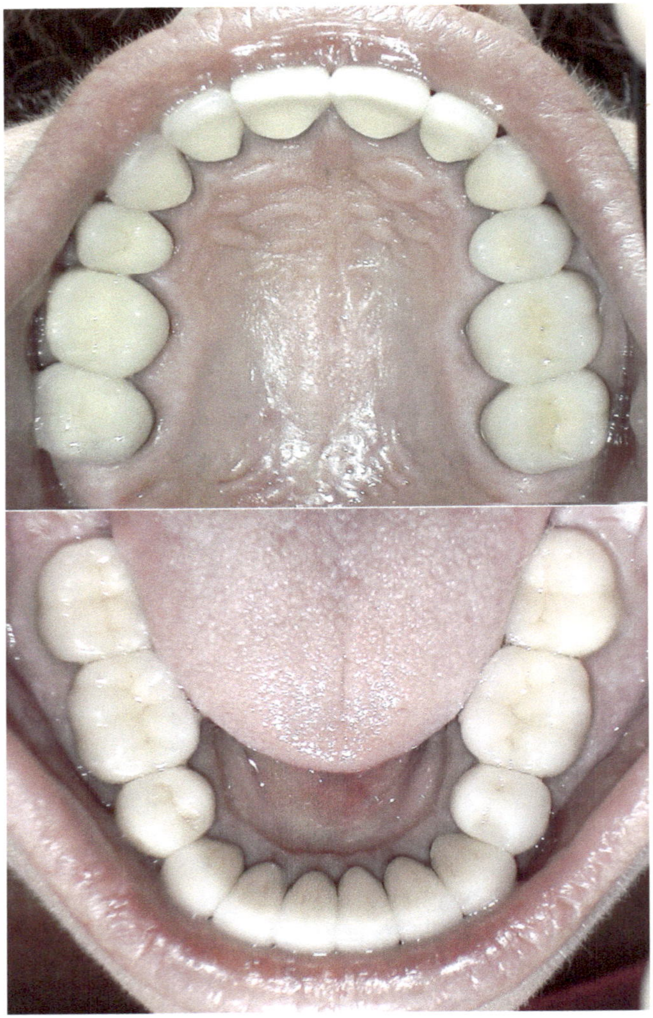

*Full Mouth Porcelain Reconstruction*

# Write Me Some Lines

*for a visiting emergency patient*

A patient who said just to tease
While I fixed his teeth up, Sir, please,
Write me a few lines
Mid the groans and the whines
For you, Sir, it should be a breeze.

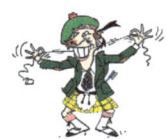

# Front Teeth - Bridges and Implants

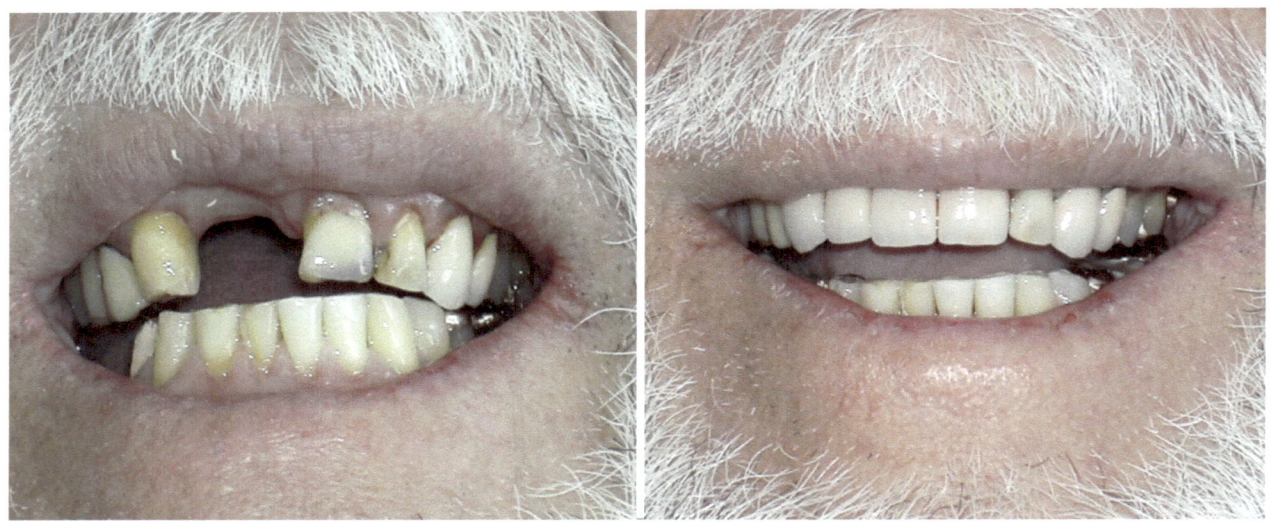

*The two missing front teeth have been replaced with a four unit bridge*

Missing teeth impair function, making eating difficult and disfigure the smile.

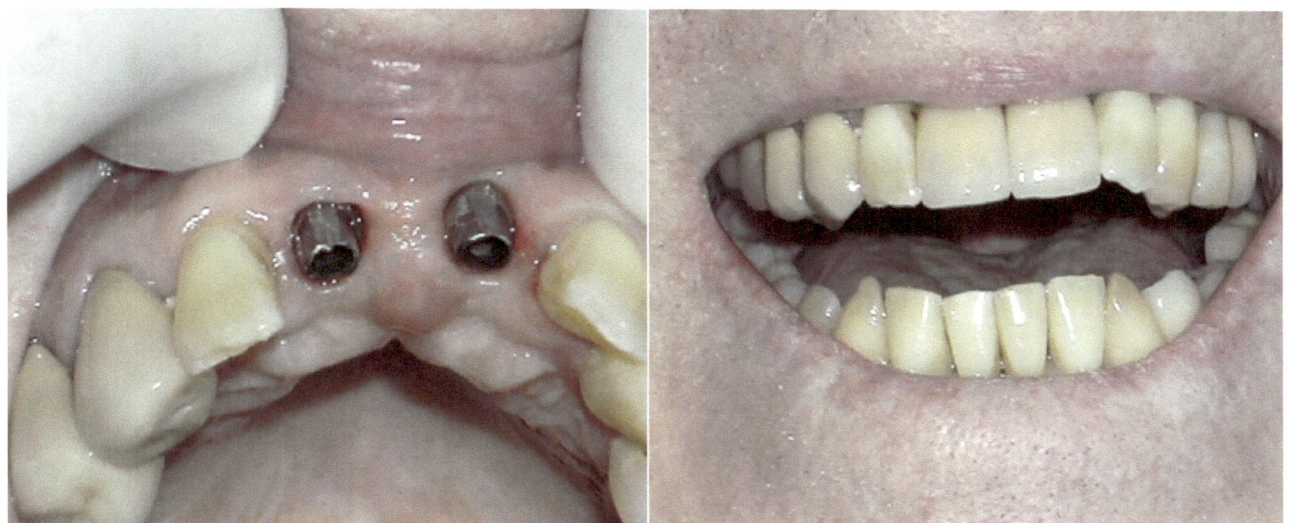

*Implants can be used to replace missing teeth*

Where enough bone is present, missing teeth are replaced with implants. The results are long lasting and look and feel absolutely natural. If bone is lacking, it is usually possible to graft additional bone before placing implants.

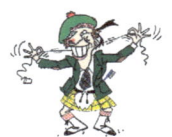

# Implants for Missing Teeth

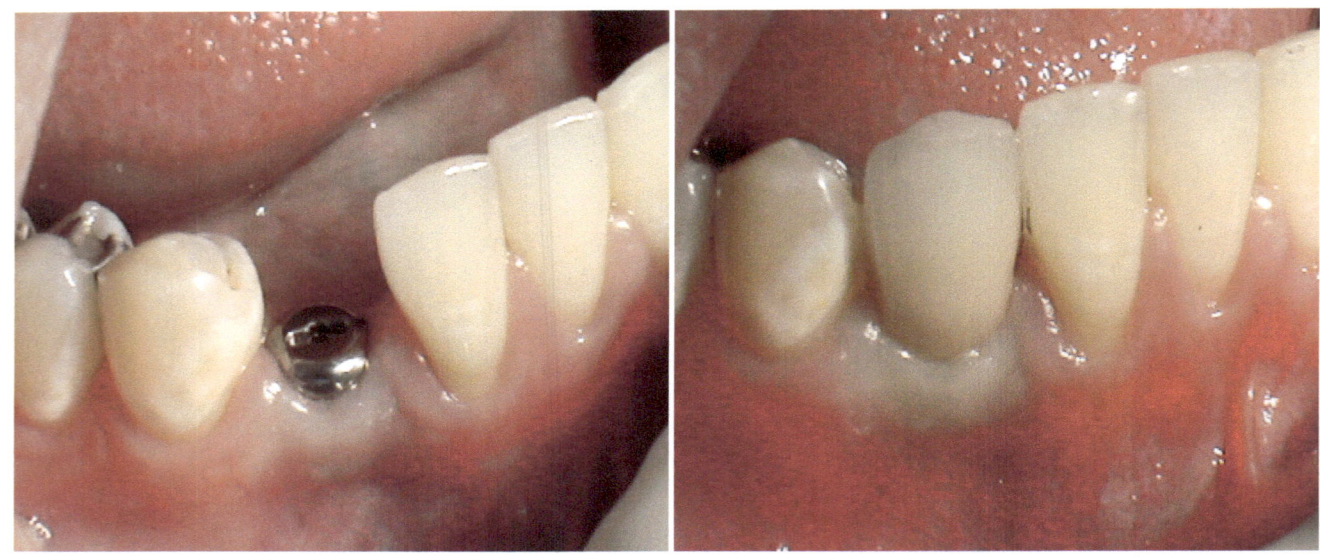

*Implant supported crown replacing a missing lower eye tooth*

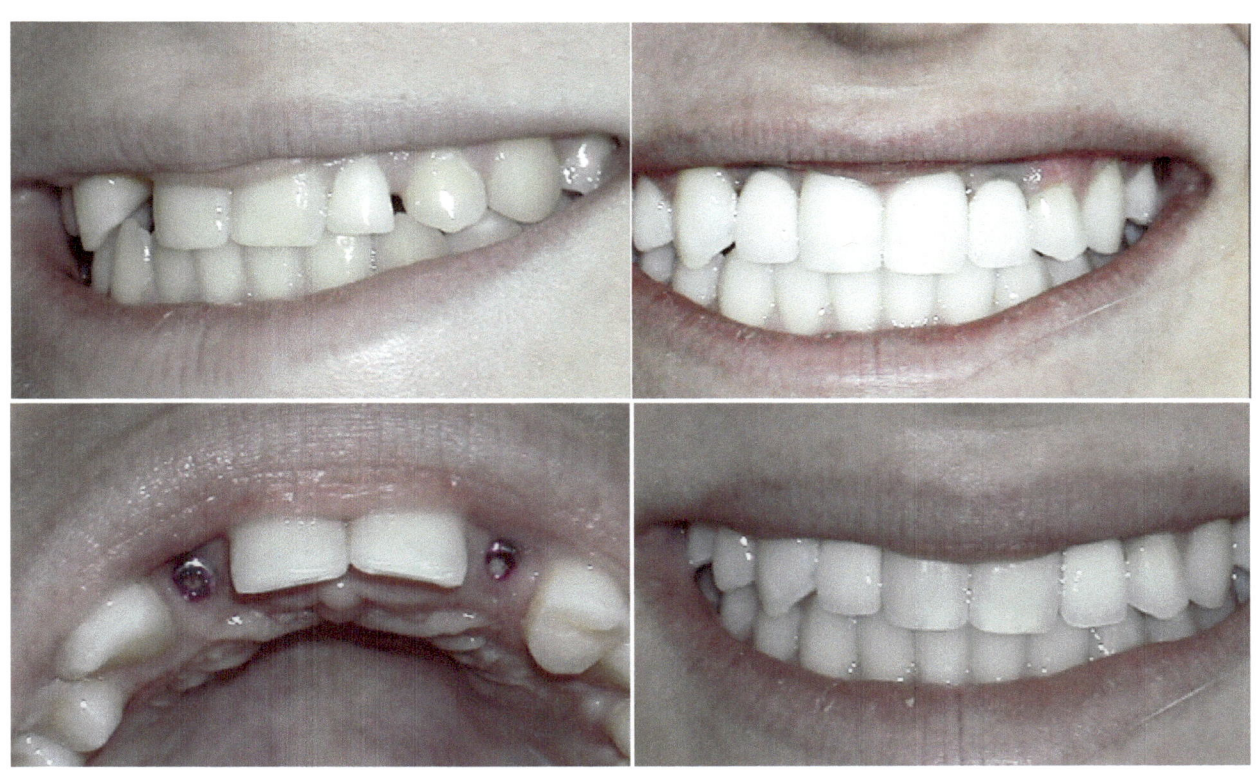

*Missing front teeth replaced with implants*

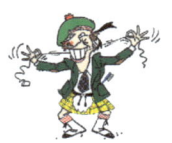

# Implant Reconstruction

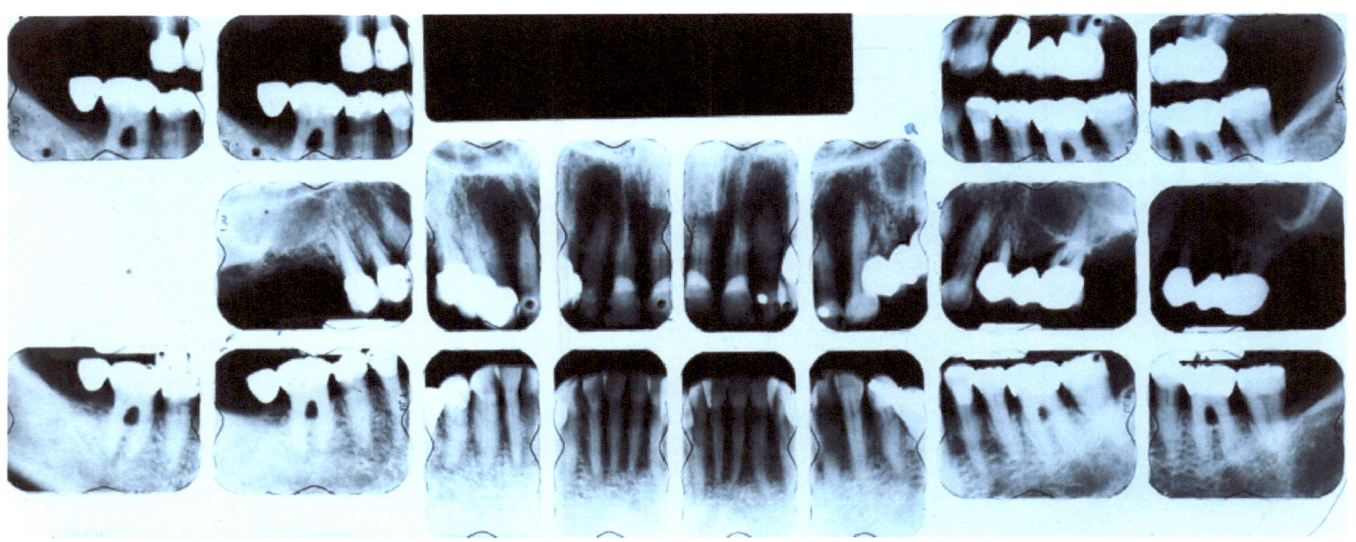

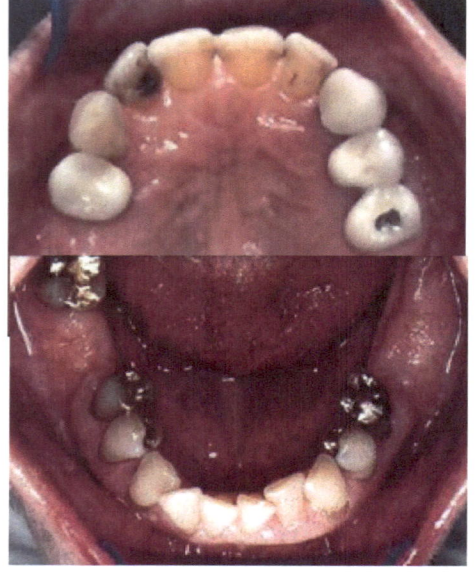

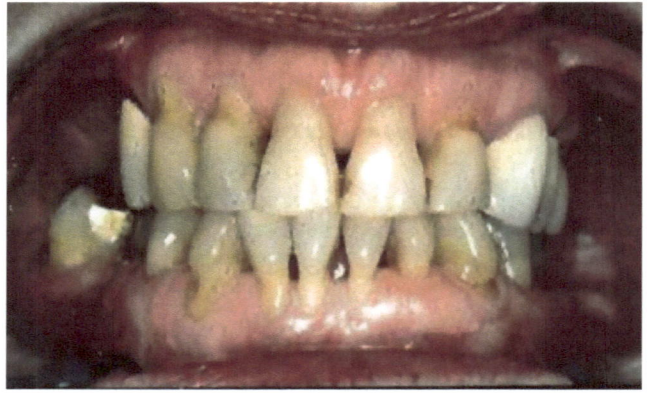

A smoker, who had lost her back teeth, quit the habit and allowed us to restore her mouth with implants and crowns.

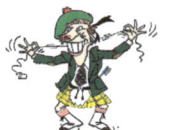

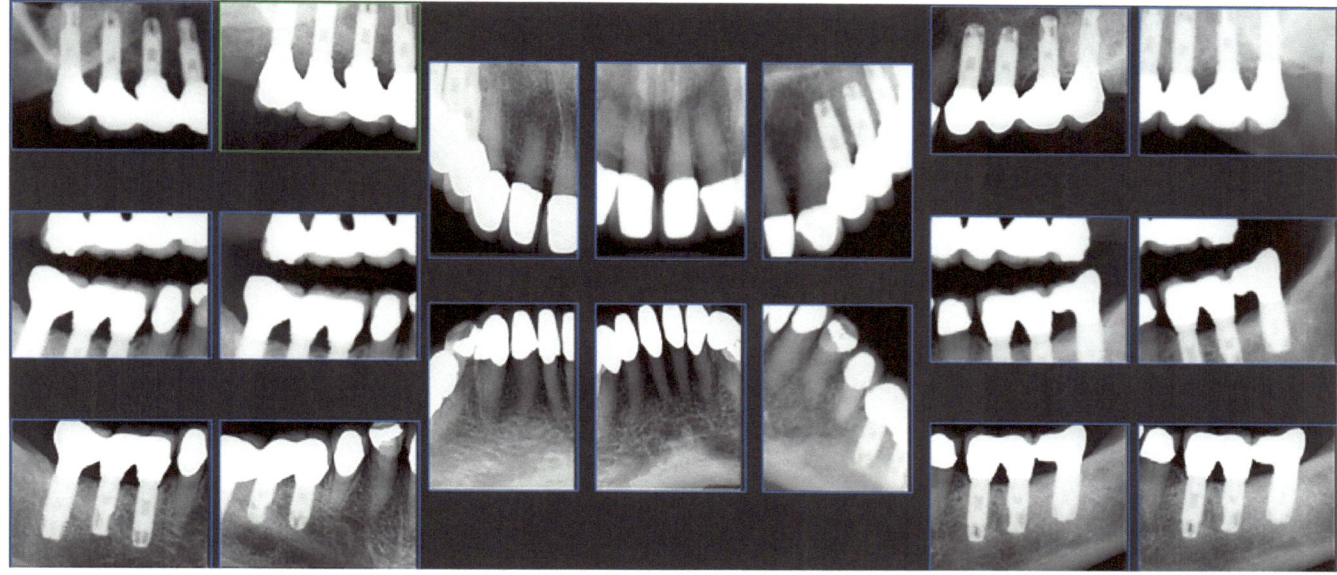

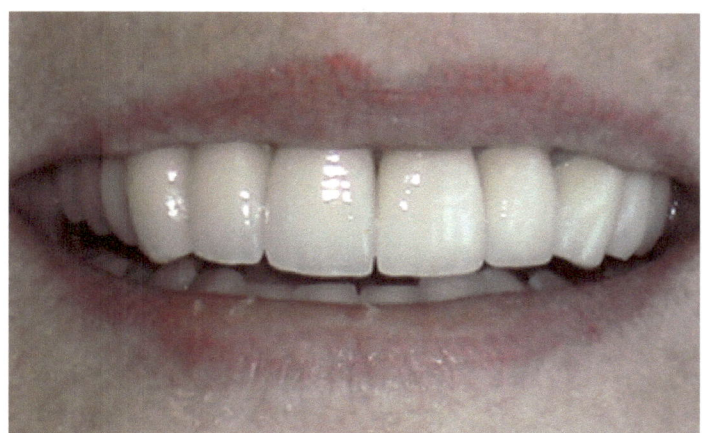
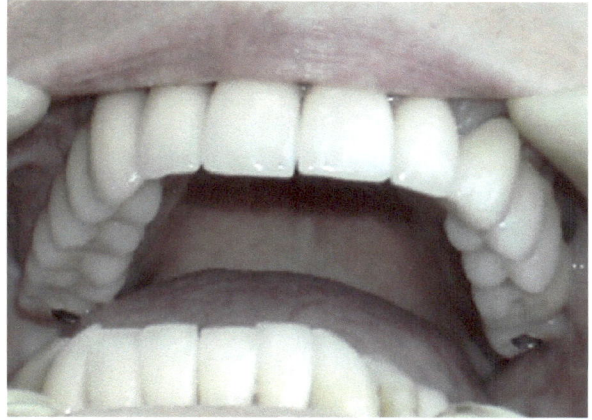

Sixteen years later the work looks like it went in yesterday. Sinus lifts were performed to develop the bone necessary to support the implants in the upper jaw.

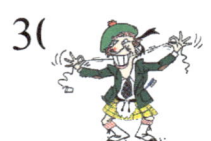

# Teeth Whitening

It seems as if everyone wants to have a whiter smile. We can help you achieve that and enhance your image. We never guarantee the results because every patient is different. We do consistently get pleasing results which enhances self esteem.

Here is an example of the Zoom Whitening™ in process.

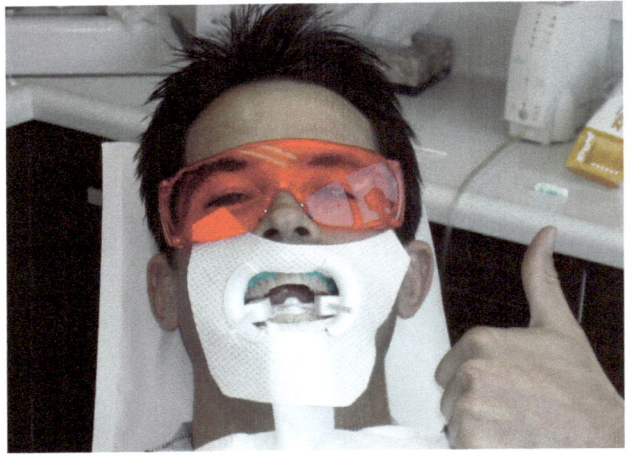

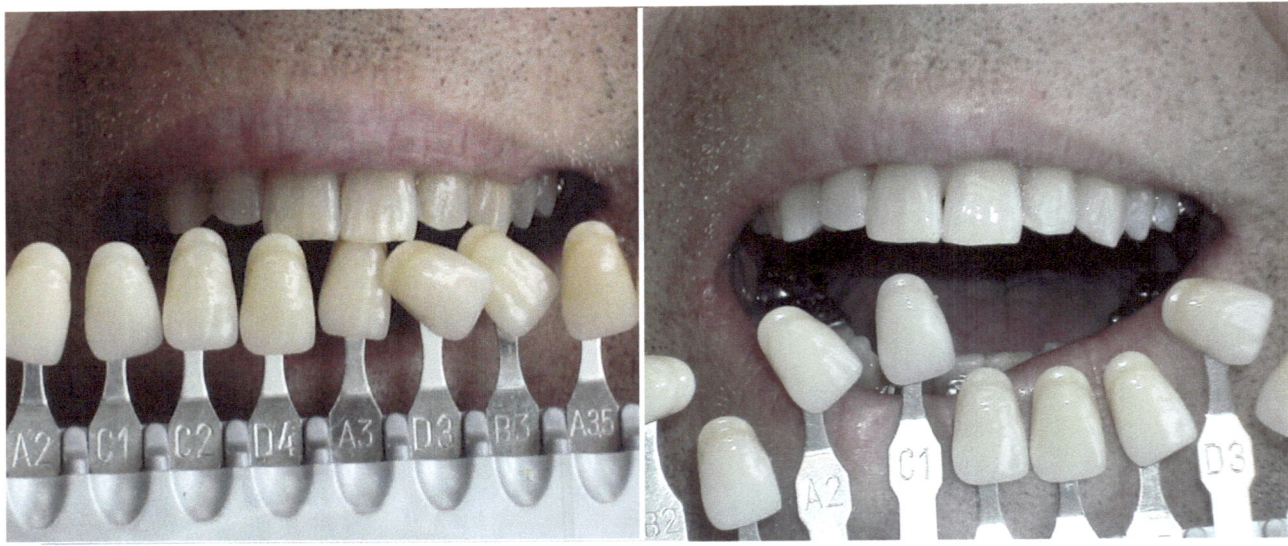

*A shift from A3 to C1 is a 3shade lightening*

# Veneers

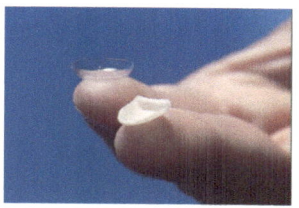

Nearly egg shell thin, but with tremendous strength, veneers can be used to cover up a multitude of defects and make a smile look beautiful.

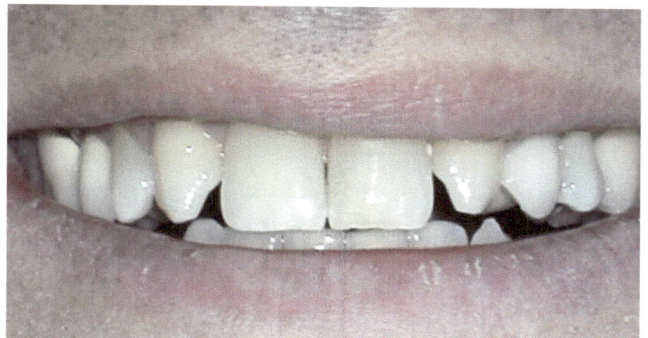

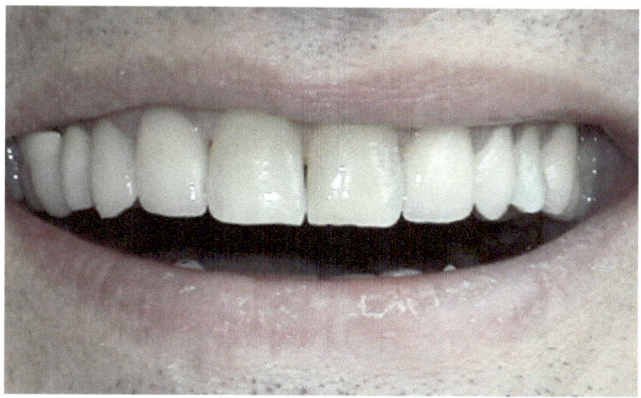

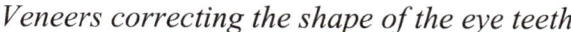

*Veneers correcting the shape of the eye teeth*

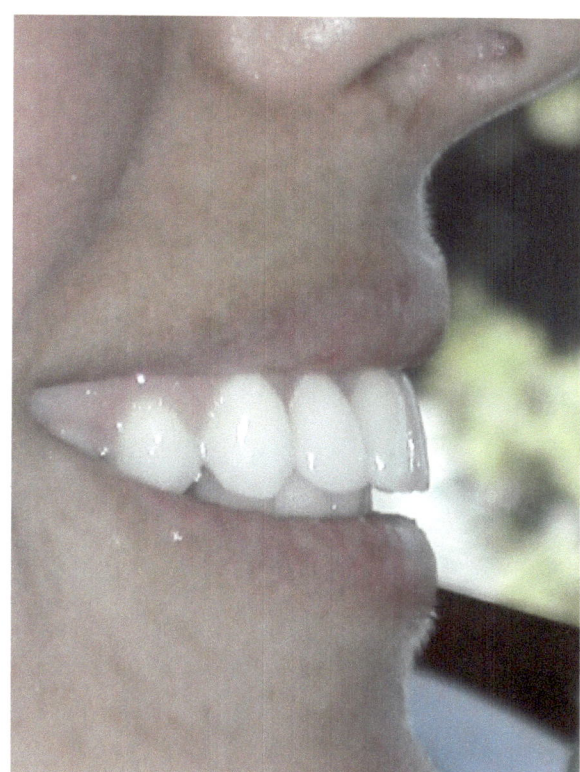

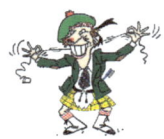

# Partial Dentures and Full Dentures

We replace missing teeth with removable partial or complete dentures, so essential to restore chewing efficiency and esthetics. At first glance you would not even realize how many teeth are being replaced. But this patient only has four upper teeth and six in the lower jaw. The partial dentures here are made out of acrylic and have wrought wire clasps. They are transitional and are worn while the patient is prepared for implant supported crowns.

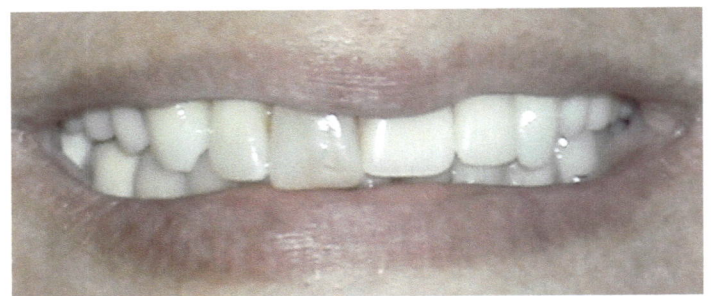

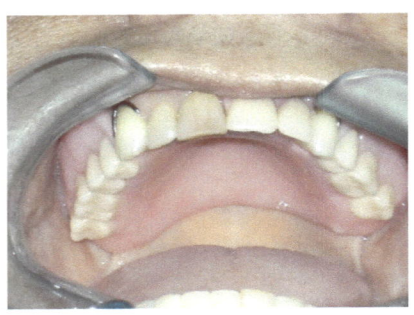
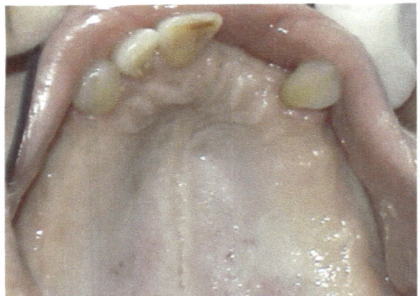
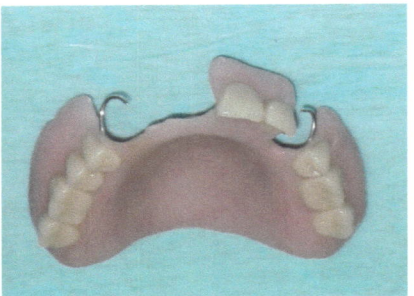

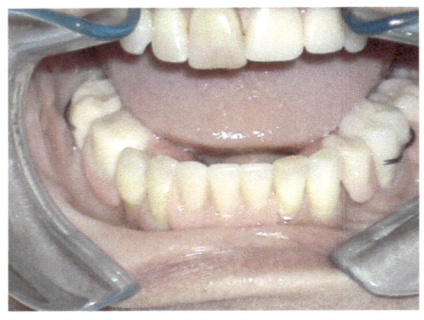
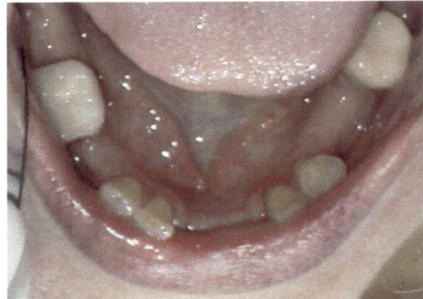
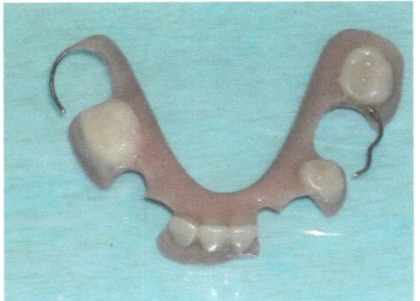

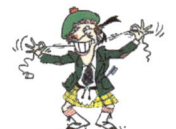 

# Precision Attachments

Partial dentures or removable bridges which sounds a little more attractive, are held in place with clasps which often show in the smile. A more precise way of connecting removable dental bridges and partials is with precision attachments which have a number of advantages one of which is that clasps do not show in the smile.

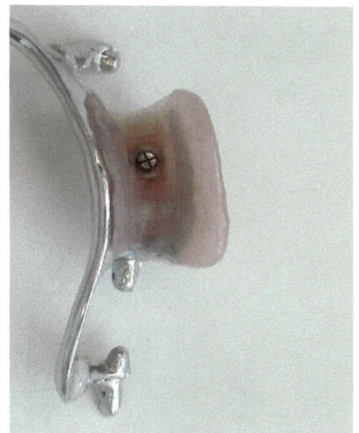

*Fitting surface showing the attachment*

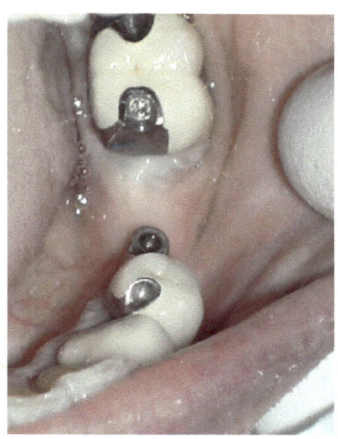

*Crowns showing rests and attachment seats*

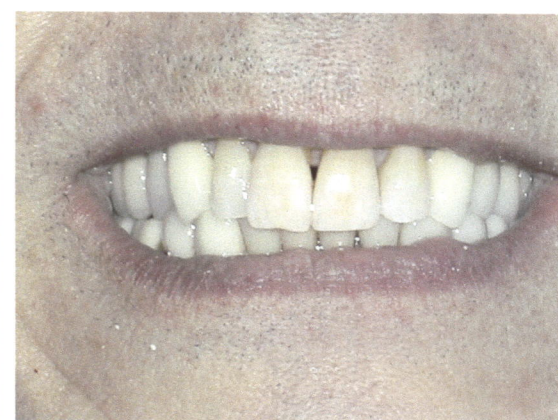

*Smile with no visible clasps*

Implants are a wonderful innovation, we use them in dentistry to replace missing teeth. For those who do not want implants, or do not have the bone to place implants the precision attachment partial is often and extremely viable alternative. It is possible to make partial dentures that do not show in the smile, which can restore the function of the mouth. Furthermore, it is possible to design and provide such treatments in a month. A great time saving. Remember, implants frequently require bone grafts to support them which take three months to organize into solid bone, and then the implant itself can take three to six months to integrate before it can be finally restored.

Precision attachments are an excellent alternative if you have some well supported teeth to which the partials can be connected.

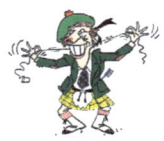

Ceka Precision Attachment retained, gold framed upper detachable bridge engineered by Swiss Quality Dental Ceramics.

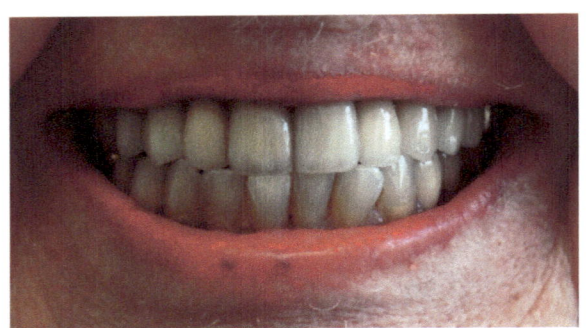

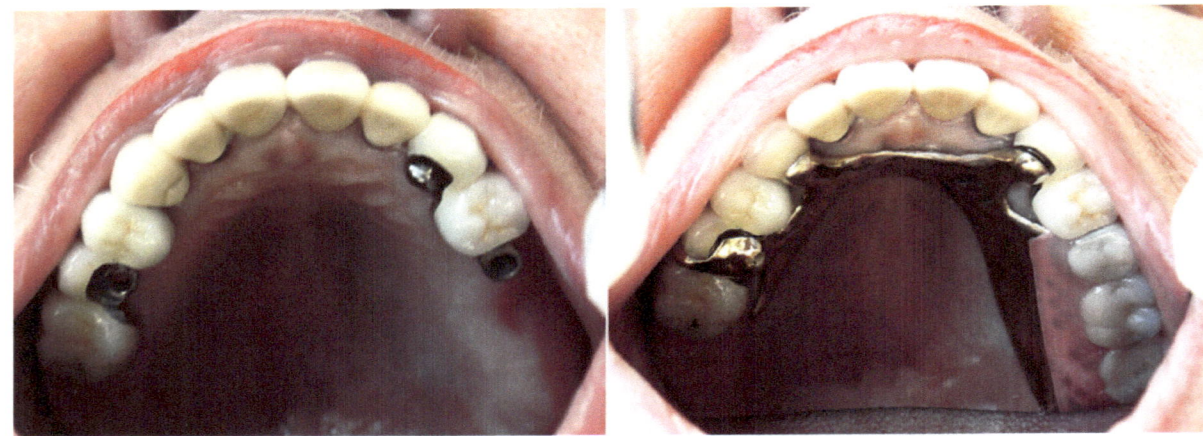

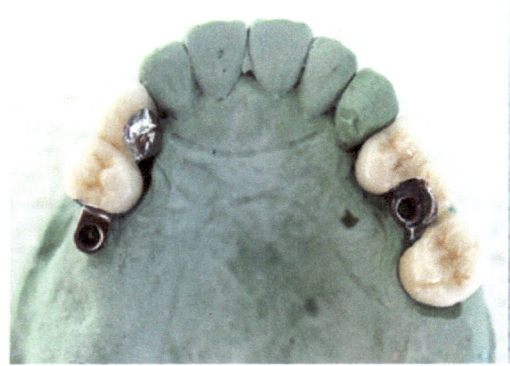
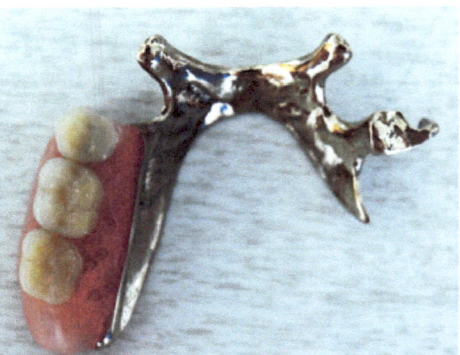
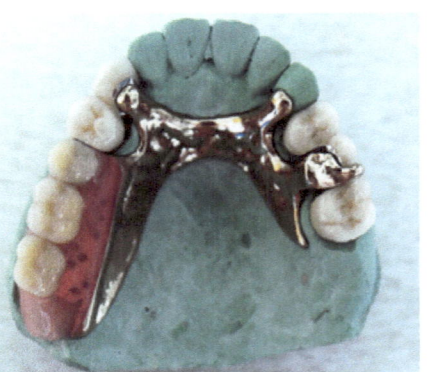

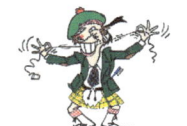

# George Washington's Teeth
## and other misconceptions

For years I have been correcting people who say that George Washington's teeth were made of wood. They were not. They were carved in ivory by John Greenwood, his Philadelphia dentist. Cleaning them during the campaign was difficult so he soaked them in port wine which stopped them from smelling and made them taste better. The port wine stained the natural grain of the elephant dentine and bone making them look wooden. Michelangelo Buonarroti, the extraordinary Italian sculptor and painter, contrary to the widely pervasive myth, did not fresco the ceiling of the Sistine Chapel lying on his back. It is a mistranslation of Paolo Giovio, the Bishop of Nocera's "Michaelis Angeli Vita" where he used "resupinus" which means "bent backwards" and not as it has been erroneously translated "on his back". Then of course there is Newton's Apple. The Universal Laws of Gravitation did not occur to Newton after an apple had fallen on his head as he was gazing up at the moon. But there may be a grain of truth in the notion that seeing an apple fall started him asking why. In "Pricipia" he discusses the effect of objects falling under gravity.

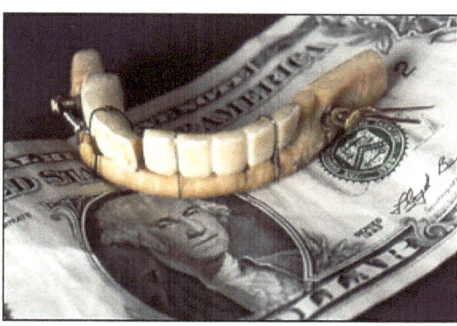

# Misconceptions

Misconceptions so often prevail,
They rob us of honest detail,
They clutter the mind,
With notions that bind,
Of the cleverest female or male.

We really should root them all out,
Removing the reason to doubt,
That the tales we are told
By the young and the old
Are really worth bandying about.

To tell you the truth I despair
At the apple that fell through the air,
And struck Isaac's head
Releasing the thread
Of the theory of gravity there.

When Washington's dentures you view
It's simply not right to construe
That they're made out of wood
For wood is no good
That popular myth is not true.

Michelangelo, its widely known,
Lay on his back 'neath the dome
Of the Sistine to paint
Well that's something that ain't,
So the next time you hear it please moan!

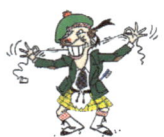

# Full Dentures

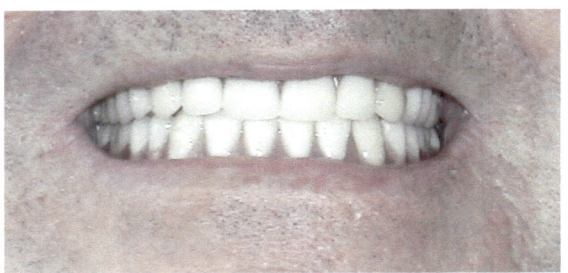

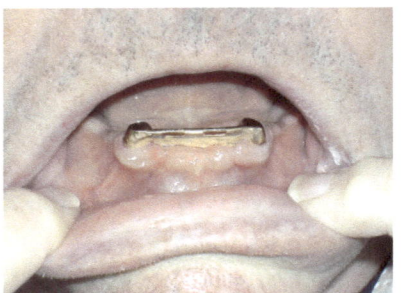

*True or False?*

Well made dentures should be hard to detect. It should be comfortable to eat with them. Lower dentures are commonly more loose than uppers, and it is invaluable to have at least a couple of teeth left which can be used to retain them. Here a gold bar is used so that clips can hold the denture down.

We have come a long way since the time when we used to set fallen soldiers' teeth into carved ivory or bone bases with pins to make dentures for the wealthy. They were called "Waterloo Teeth".

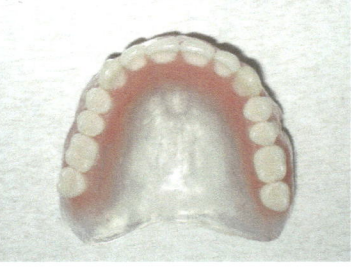

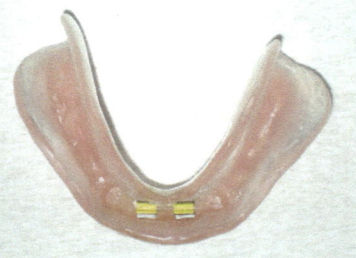

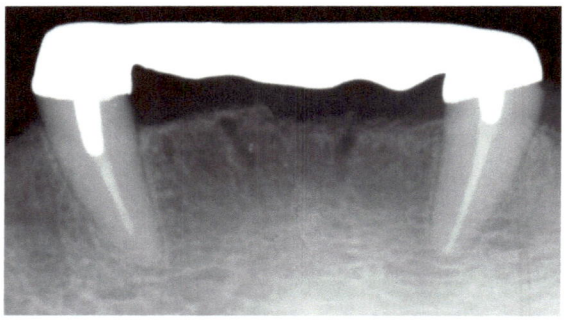

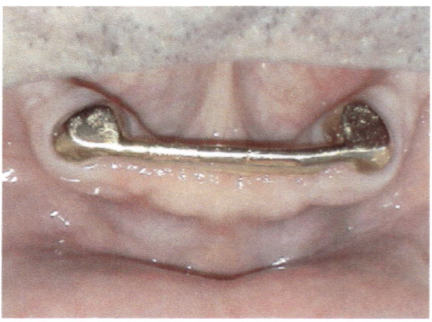

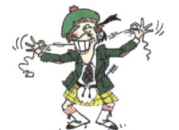 

# Root Canal Treatments and Posts

Decay, fractures, trauma, clenching and exposure to excessive temperature extremes can all cause the nerve within the tooth to die. When that happens, the patient needs root canal therapy. In the absence of the blood vessels and nerves the tooth gradually gets more brittle and around the seventh year may no longer be able to withstand the pressure of the bite. These teeth need to be reinforced with strong posts to transfer the force into a part of the tooth structure supported in the bone. It is the firm belief in this practice that a properly made gold post and core build ups are still the best way the restore such teeth.

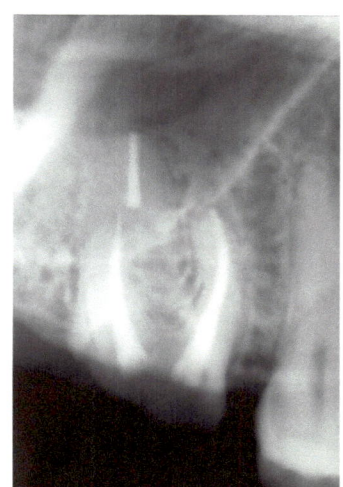

*Root Treatment*

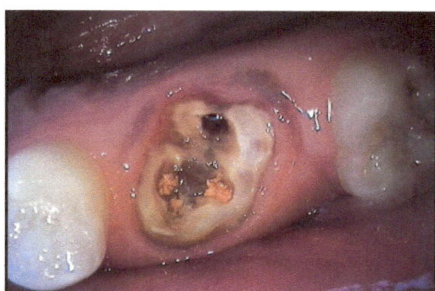

*Seriously broken down molar*

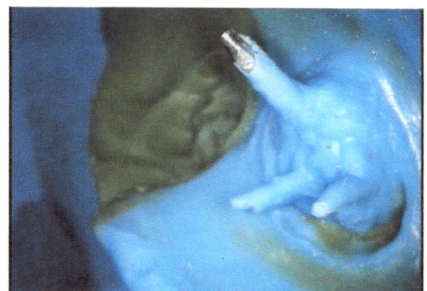

*The impression*

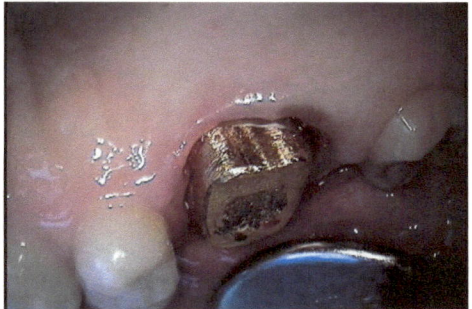

*Restored ready for a crown*

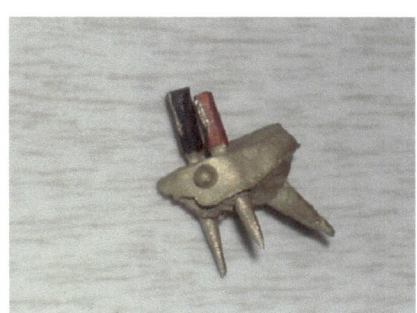

*Triple interlocked post*

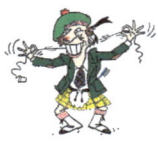

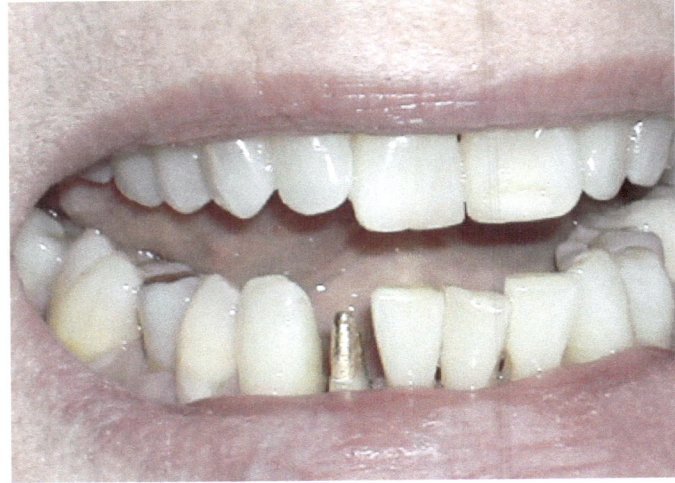

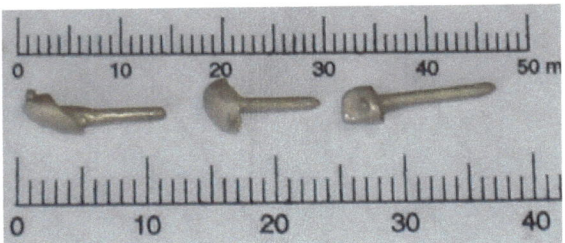

Posts need to be long enough to conduct the biting force into a part of the root of the tooth that is supported by strong bone.

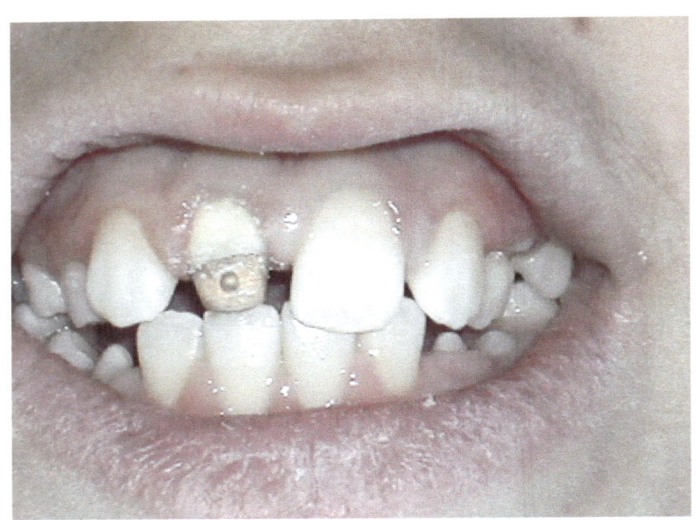

*Broken teeth restored with gold posts*

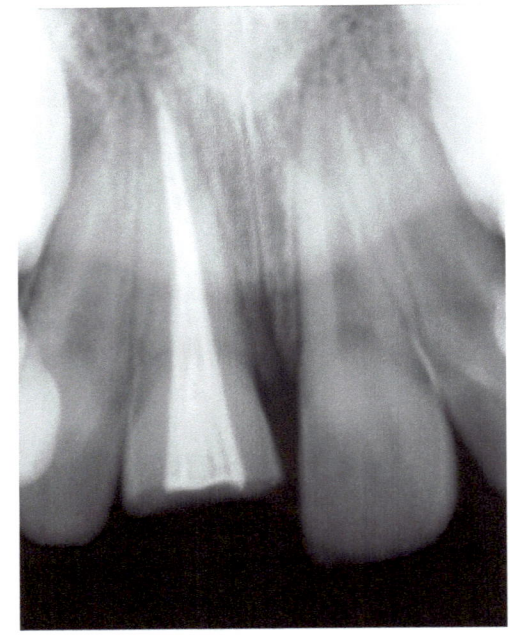

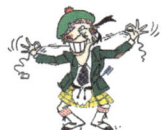

# Bite Guards and Sports Guards

These are two very different preventative aids. The bite guard, properly called an occlusal guard, prevents you from grinding your teeth away and prevents you putting undue pressure on the teeth when clenching them.

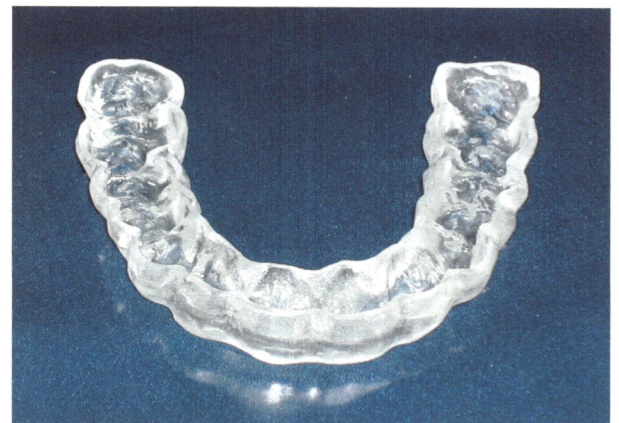

*Classic contoured hard acrylic "Night Guard"*

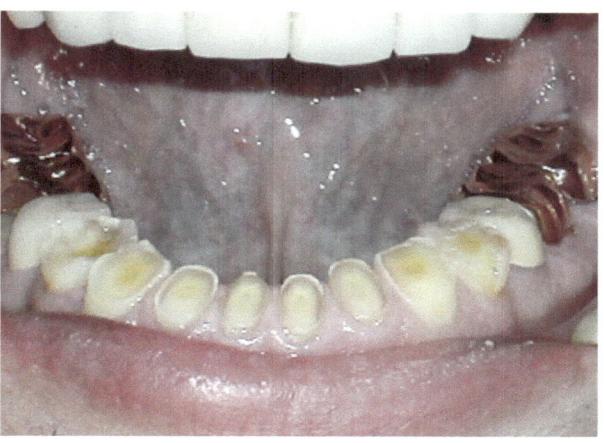

*Excessive erosion and grinding*

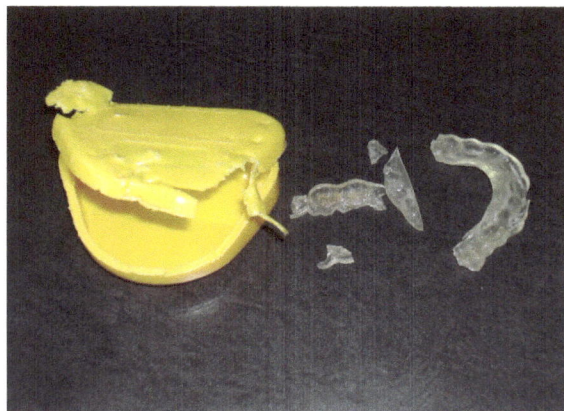

*Pets love them!*

## About Hank

A Lab Man, who answered to Hank,
Had a dentist he wanted to thank,
So he scrawled a few lines
With some most obscure rhymes
And signed Socrates just to add rank.

His mouth guards fit well, to be frank,
So his business is not "in the tank,"
He churns out acrylic
While writing a lyric,
And laughs all the way to the bank.

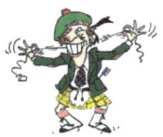

The sports guard is an impact absorbing shield engineered to stop you from chipping or knocking your teeth out when participating in contact sports. They are not worn enough, and records indicate that a million teeth are knocked out every year by athletes not wearing them.

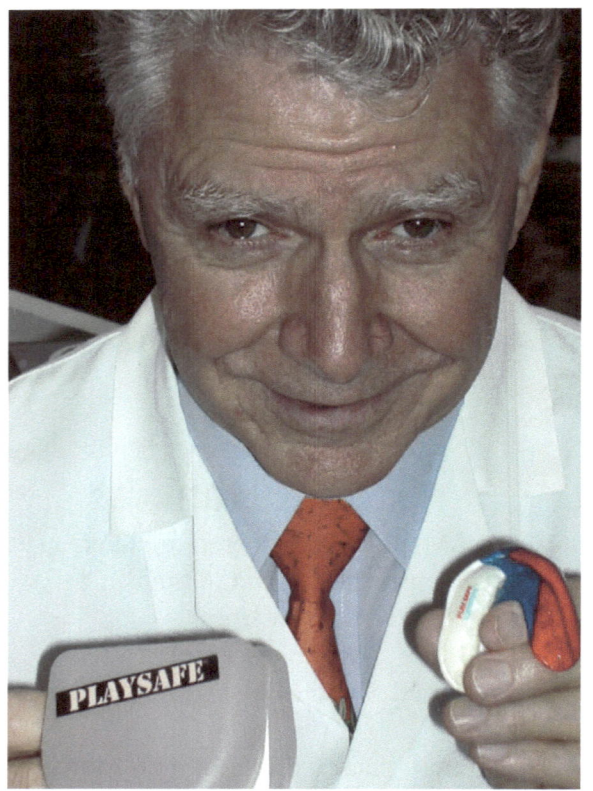

*Close fitting vacuum molded athletic and contact Sports Guard*

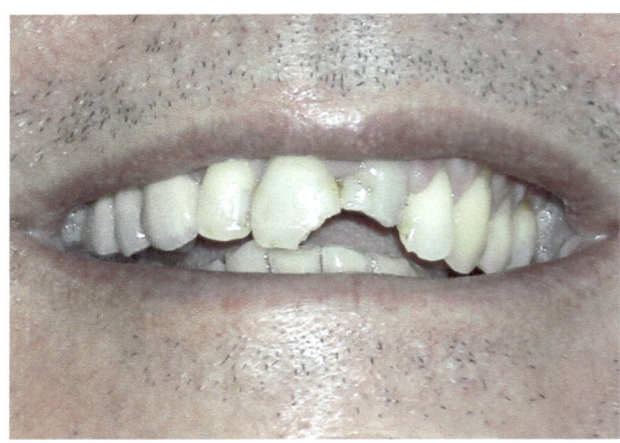

*A sports guard might have prevented this*

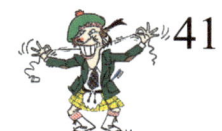

# Bruxism - Tooth Grinding

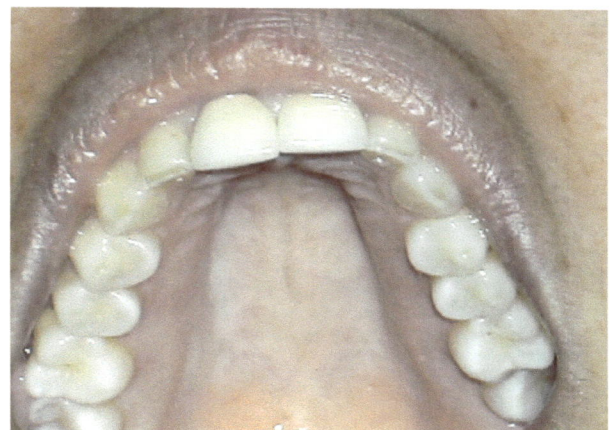

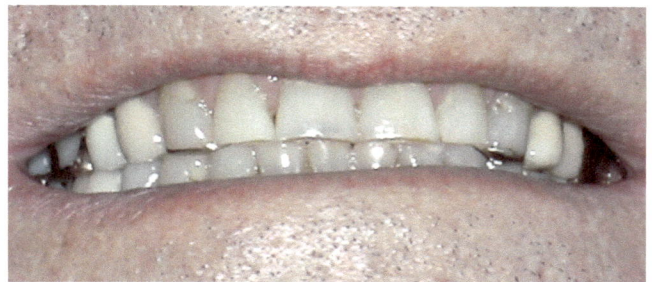

*Classic worn teeth of a Bruxer*

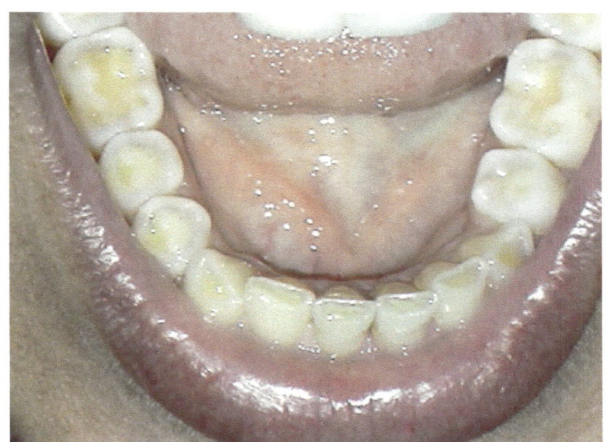

*Bruxing and erosion*

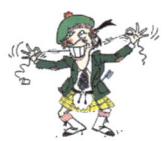

# Tooth Straightening

Misaligned teeth generally become more irregular with time making them more difficult to clean and more likely to be affected by bone loss. Crooked teeth often contributes to a sense of low self esteem. By wearing appliances which are removable for eighteen hours a day some remarkable improvements can be achieved. The development of aligning trays has made the process even easier.

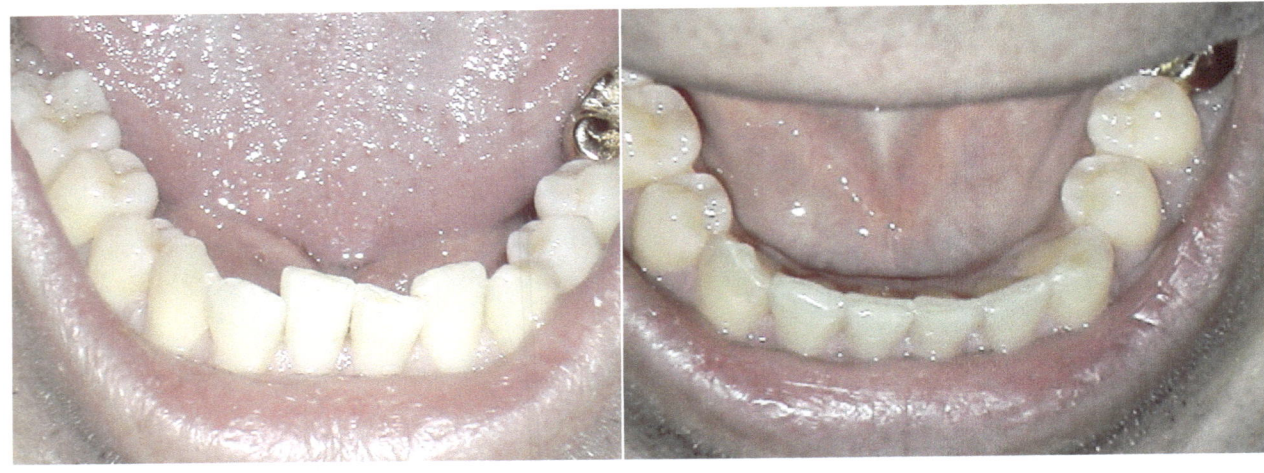

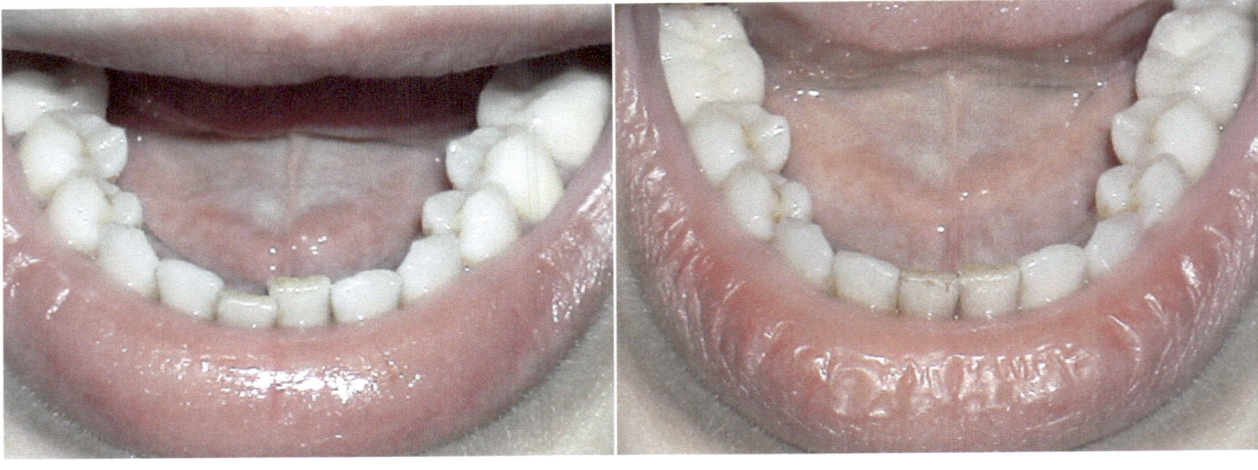

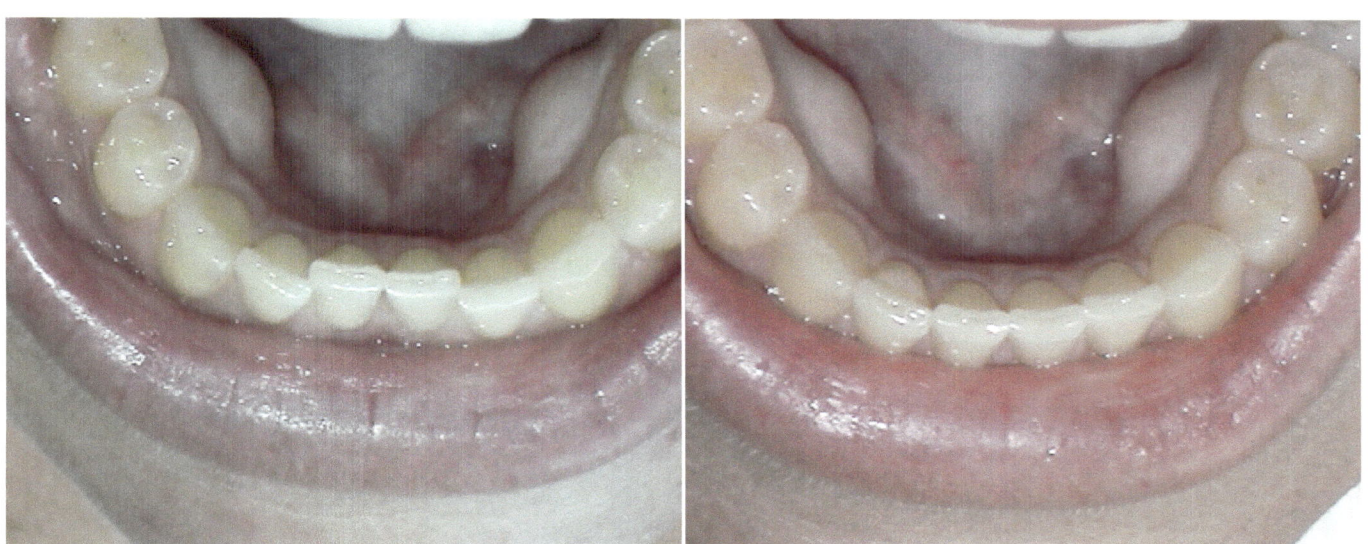

## How To Squeeze

*When you share toothpaste in a family it is a drag to have to flatten out the tube every time you want to express your little dab of paste. Inevitably, someone else has squeezed in the middle and messed it up. Small potatoes Huh!*

When you squeeze the toothpaste tube
Please squeeze it from the bottom,
If you use another way
You're doing something rotten.

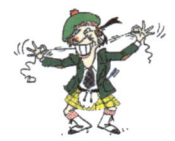

Please Father!

I will try to do better,
I'll try to keep my socks pulled up,
I'll watch where I'm going in future,
And not sit down in the muck.
I know that my jersey's in tatters,
My white mouse, he nibbled the thread
So he can peek out during lessons,
And get some fresh air round his head.
I know that my shoes are all scuffed up
I'm getting some polish next week,
My Mum's coming round at half term,
I'm excited, that's really a treat.

Please Father!
I will try to do better,
I've washed hands, see nails free of loam,
The curls on my head just will not lie flat,
Since last week when I lost my comb.
My "S" belt it seems to be missing,
I looked for a long time last night,
The boy in the next bed may've nicked it,
Cause I flicked him and gave him a fright.
I do brush my teeth every morning,
I try not to miss when it's late,
Mum say's if I don't she must take me
To the dentist, something I will hate.

# Fractured Teeth

We can be deceived into thinking our teeth are as strong as nails, especially when we're young, but they can be cracked and broken quite easily. Even a small tap against a cup or bottle, or the edge of a pool, can do serious damage that can last and affect you for a lifetime. You can even break a tooth by biting down on something hard, or just by clenching your teeth together with enough force. Let us not forget that silver fillings can crack teeth because of the rate at which they expand with temperature change due to the mercury content.

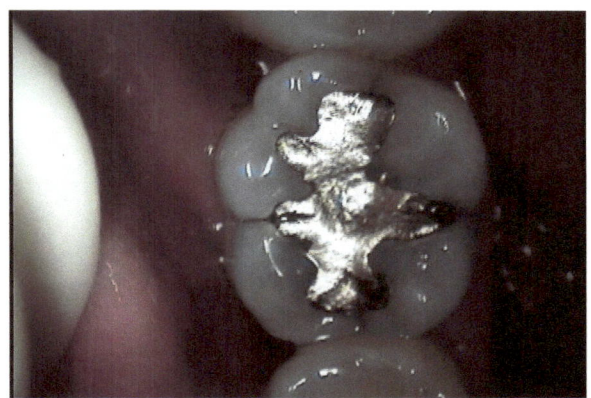
*Alloy filling has cracked the tooth*

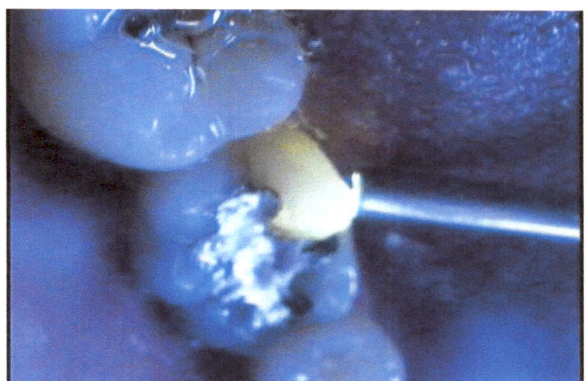
*Fiber optically illuminated fracture*

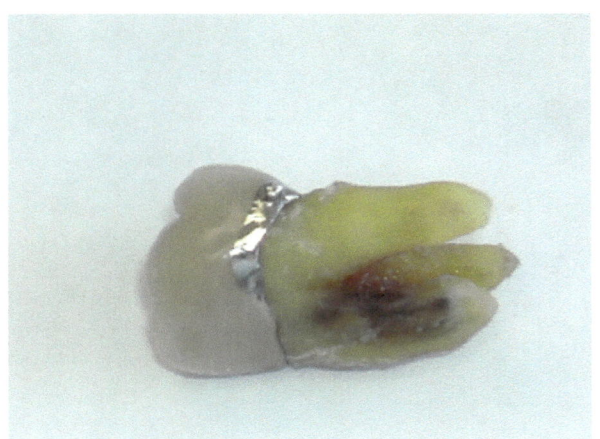
*Failed molar with fractured root*

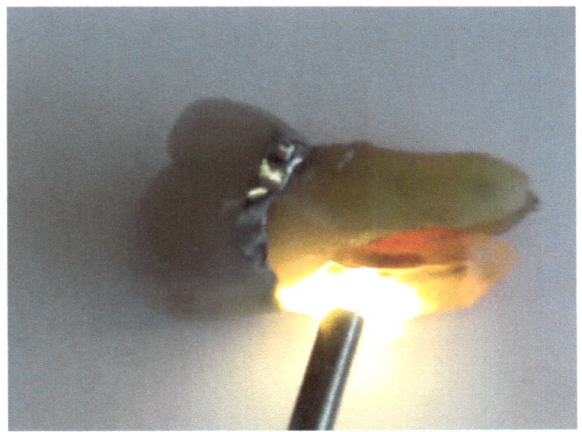
*Fiber optically illuminated root crack*

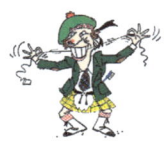

# The Staff

This practice could not exist without the support of well-qualified continually-educated and competent staff. Over the last four decades, there have been changes but, looking back, thanks are due to Liz Mineo, Karen Greenhouse, Freddie Fink, Marsha Nicholas and Carole Paramor who have all been front desk office managers. Many wonderful assistants have come and gone too. Mercifully "Sandy" is still on team loyal and true completing our present staff who are equal to the task.

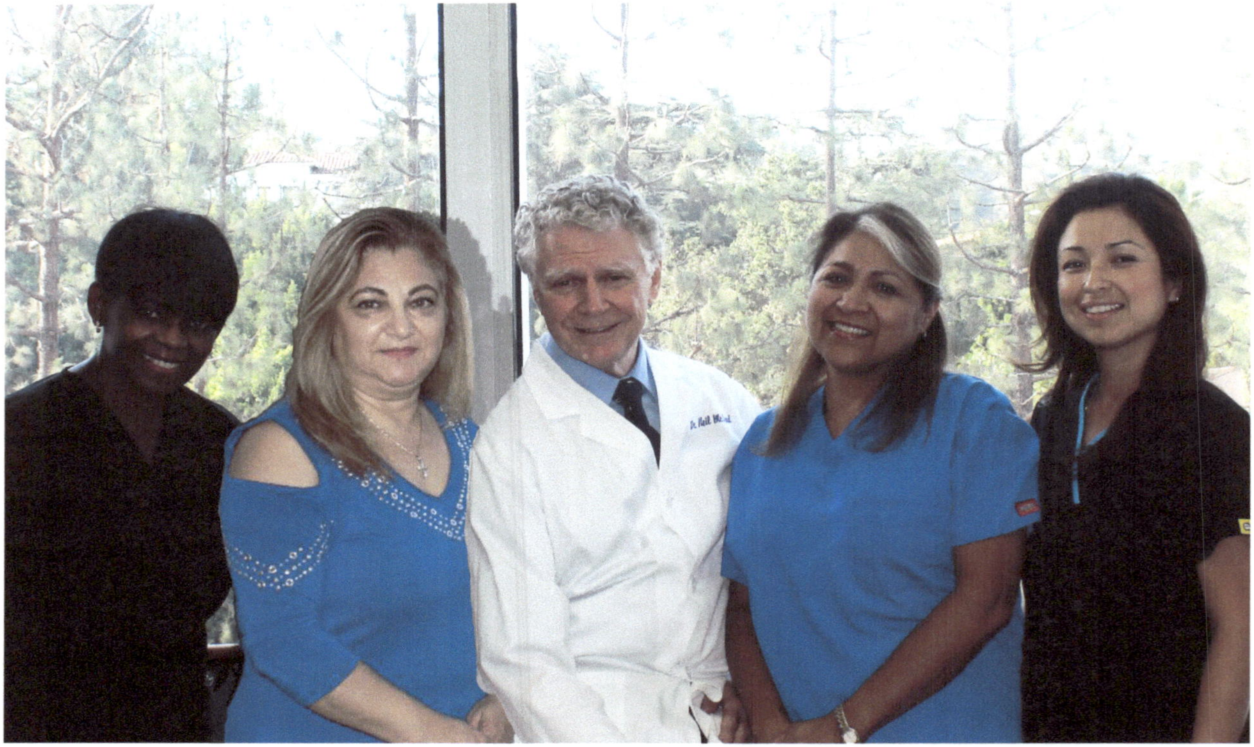

*Darlene Hitchins RDH , Maral Merzoian RDA,  Dr.Neil McLeod DDS, ,Sandra Bischof RDA, Mayra Pool RDH*

# Acknowledgments

Special thanks must be expressed to all the patients who have trusted us to care for them over the years, and whose images form the basis of the examples displayed on these pages, and also to our professional colleagues, the specialist with whom we work and to whom we refer our patients when the finest specialty treatments are required to achiev the best results. Anne Talltree must be thanked for her editorial eye.

Neil Stewart McLeod
Los Angeles 2019

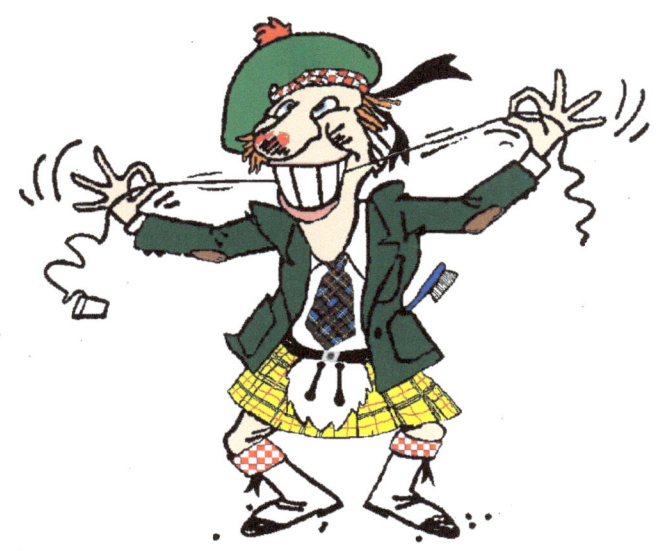

*Phil MaCavity says "Just floss 'em!*